Billy's
MONSTER

A Love and Life Surrendered Amidst War
With the Alzheimer's Monster

Lisa Filler

Kick in the Pants Bookworks

DEDICATION

For Levi and Autumn.
For those who wrote themselves into our story.
For the kind professionals who guided me and calmed the panic.
And for all of those who loved my Billy and rallied from the sidelines.

Thank you.

TABLE OF CONTENTS

INTRODUCTION

THE EARLY YEARS of my life were rooted in the center of a close-knit family in central Montana, until I met and married my Billy Filler. I immersed myself in the treasured duties of wife and mother before a diagnosis of early-onset Alzheimer's disease stopped us in our tracks. An overwhelming desire to document the relentless ravages of this unyielding disease soon became my prescription for strength.

Our story details a surreal and adventure-filled, three-year final season alongside Billy, my once strong-willed and independent husband, diagnosed with early-onset Alzheimer's disease at the age of fifty-four. Shortly after his initial diagnosis, I uprooted our life in rural Montana and transplanted it on the serene Oregon coast, a few hours from Billy's mother and his brother, and where we had also frolicked with our children for a few glorious days nearly every summer since we married. Our new world, I termed *Our Bubble at the Beach*, was surreal and finite, a whirlwind of events cut short by Billy's inevitable defeat by his insidious monster. My new world proved both heart-wrenching and rewarding when I found myself a helpless spectator on the sidelines of his escalating nightmare. Spiritual growth and maturity were continual by-products of releasing the reins of a planned out future and free-falling through clouds of the unknown, fully aware of the painful impact that could occur at any given moment.

Early-onset Alzheimer's without a genetic component itself is quite rare, but a twist in the last days of our journey revealed a possible and yet rarer diagnosis of Multiple System Atrophy, which left hindsight of many unusual symptoms popping in and out of my mind in the months that followed Billy's transition from the physical to the spiritual world.

Alzheimer's disease has become a research priority and has been deemed an epidemic in many articles, and Billy's brain and spinal cord are now in the hands of research scientists. I am hopeful that someday in the near future their hard work will eliminate for others the horrors my Billy and so many others have already endured. Interest and awareness is also on the rise and I hope our story will inspire the courage necessary to face one day at a time for anyone searching for answers throughout the same dark tunnels. A newly acquired awareness of the lack of support for the mentally impaired has left my naïve spirit bruised, and though I have found solace in documenting our story, I am also hopeful that should it find its way into the hands of readers enduring the same complex tragedy, it may prepare them in advance and inspire courage to seek God's grace and presence where they would least expect it.

CHAPTER 1

SEASONS

MELANCHOLY AND APPREHENSION snuck up next to me that crisp fall afternoon, forcing me to snuggle deep into Billy's warm shoulder when a reminder of our grim future pushed unwelcome tears through my squinted lashes. The October sun danced wildly between fragrant pine boughs bobbing to and fro in the cool Pacific breeze, drying my damp cheeks and easing me into a spirit of gratefulness for the perfect moment enveloping us. I slid over the rough and weathered picnic bench, leaning even deeper into the softness of his Oregon Ducks pullover while bits of autumn's gold swirled into lyrics of old rock tunes that were banging out from atop a rusty flatbed trailer.

My gaze settled onto a free spirit draped in a long colorful halter dress, arms outstretched as if saluting the golden sun, and swaying seductively to the music of an era she so clearly missed. We sipped our frosty brew and absorbed the nostalgia floating gently through the eclectic crowd that had followed the free spirit onto the dusty dance floor. That *Artoberfest* on the Oregon Coast, a community gathering to celebrate the season, handcrafted beer, and the artistic spirit, would be the grand finale of the very significant summer that had so swiftly slipped by.

The world as we knew it ended on a cold January morning in Montana when the official diagnosis of early-onset Alzheimer's disease for my Billy, at the young age of fifty-four, dashed all of our hopes that his forgetfulness and fatigue were due to long hours of work and stress. The only consolation was that we now knew the name of the monster banging at our door. That monster, lurking slyly in the shadows at first, had become quite obnoxious by the time Billy agreed to an appointment with a neurologist.

It wasn't long before an observant and thorough specialist reviewed an MRI of Billy's brain from the year prior and was shocked by the abnormal and generalized atrophy it revealed. Unfortunately, we had been assured during those earlier rounds of poking and prodding, in hopes of discoveries to strange symptoms, that nothing abnormal was present and we should consider treatment for depression. A new and immediate battery of exhausting mental exams and weeks of patiently waiting for spinal tap fluid results dismissed the assumption of a possible chemical imbalance, along with the previous doctor's haphazard guess at depression. Once all reports were in, the nurse practitioner assigned to our case was finally prepared to give our insidious monster its name.

It was cold outside. My cells ached with winter's chill, and anxiety slowly increased, along with the miles between Havre and Great Falls, in desperate hope of fixable answers. We were early and waited in silence. Billy flipped nervously through magazines beneath the glaring fluorescent lights while I tried to calm the shivers rattling my bones beneath the comfort of my down-filled parka. Several elderly patients hobbled in and hobbled back out, some on the elbow of a caregiver drenched in sympathy, and others all alone, struggling with their walkers or canes. I felt conspicuously out of place.

"Mr. Filler" was finally announced, and a puzzled look from Billy followed as he tossed the magazine aside and his eyes met mine. We followed the nurse into the dimly lit, gray interior of the confining *here are your answers* room.

"Please, please, please don't shut that door," I muttered to myself.

She shut that door. Claustrophobia snuck in. My eyes focused on the giant bottle of diet soda and bright red party cups she dragged in with her and pleasantly offered.

"Wasn't that stuff bad, laced with chemicals and generally bad?" I mused, "Offered to patients in a neurologist's office?"

I studied the glaring red letters mostly concealing the sugar-free concoction behind them. Her muffled words floated like puzzle pieces in the suffocating clinical air, waiting for me to pluck and comprehend them. I was still trying to sort out the ridiculousness of offering a chemical-laden beverage to neurologically impaired patients when my mind snatched the word *Alzheimer's* from the cloud of nauseating *"blah, blah, blah"* and scripted explanations void of compassion or remedy. Fifty-four years of age and this is the monster that would devour my Billy: Alzheimer's. Not the damaging effects of habitual vices indulged in since youth, not the fate-tempting daredevil antics of speed or height. Alzheimer's. At fifty-four.

I comprehended so little of her rambling by then. More *"blah, blah, blah"* bounced around in my skull and in an instant my give-a-shit was broken beyond repair. Drink the whole damn bottle of soda, doc. Live it up, suck it down, never use a crosswalk again. The random plucking of our souls from the confines of life is uncontrollable and I finally leapt into my Billy's carefree field of wild abandon. Why do epiphanies light us up just as regret casts a heavy shadow? The irony of it. At the exact moment I traded neurosis for the unrestrained desire to truly live, the chains of responsibility tightened securely around my limbs.

The latest and *only* drugs available to slow down the monster's inevitable conquest for an unpredictable period of time were discussed.

"How long will they work?" I asked.

"Who knows, a year, maybe two?" she casually replied.

I swallowed hard when I noticed Billy watching me, looking for confirmation that I could command this monster. I stood. False confidence and a forced smile squeezed past my lips.

"Okay, Billy," I squeaked out, "now we know, and people live full lives for many years."

I lied. I knew. Neurosis had led me down the research trail.

Statistics were less than comforting. I made a silent request for generosity of time from the Giver and Taker and in faith stood to assure our medical professional that we would pick up her recommended regimen of drugs and supplements, schedule a follow-up and go right ahead and face each day with a healthy dose of denial. She nodded. A professional smile dripped down her face as she ushered us out.

Through the shadows, I peered at our monster for weeks. The research trail now dragged me through tunnels of information describing clinical trials and left me depleted. Placebos, unfavorable statistics, and discontinued trials abound. We could have gone through the process of attempting to qualify, praying that he would receive the actual trial drug and not the placebo and keep a hopeful eye for positive results, while with each sunset and sunrise another precious day of sharing the present together would be lost.

Sitting in my dimly lit, cold and now claustrophobic cubicle at work one morning, I hugged my steaming coffee mug close to my aching chest and pushed hard against the new weight bearing down on my shoulders. I visualized Billy and Jazzy, our little black pug, spending the day watching television while the biting February wind angrily drifted the steadily falling snow over mounds of rugged ice, keeping them from their daily walk. Panic rolled slowly over me and held my breath prisoner when it occurred to me that all of Billy's years of loyalty to the company he had worked for, and consistent and selfless efforts he diligently made to provide for me and our two children, would wither into a distant memory, and his beautiful mind would slowly dissolve while he waited patiently every day for me to return home from work.

The moment I was chosen for the coveted government position I held in our small community I was convinced that it was a personal gift from The Giver, as the opportunity arose at the exact time we were pondering the financial struggle facing us now that both our son and our daughter were well into their college educations. But life unfolds in seasons, and I knew my season for the highest paying job I would ever hold without a college education was ending, and a season of caregiver for my sweetheart was beginning. With the words *for richer or for poorer, in sickness and in health* resonating in my mind, and fear rising up from deep within me at the mere thought of resigning from the position I had held for just a few short years, I began an online search for homes on the Oregon Coast where we had vacationed nearly every summer since our honeymoon twenty-six years ago. Real life would begin now—the life that waits patiently for enough money, enough time, retirement, chores, fears, children. Our *golden* years had begun far sooner than expected, and the nest egg my Billy had so carefully guarded would now fund the present rather than the unsure future. I left work that afternoon a little less discouraged, yet much more apprehensive, as I contemplated the next season of our life together.

I divulged my ideas to Billy after dinner, and was surprised by the instant spark of hopefulness in his eyes. He had been home alone nearly every day since November when a car accident, and the neurologist's recommendation that he no longer drive due to surprisingly poor results of preliminary tests, had required him to take a leave of absence from work until a definite diagnosis could be made. I suggested a house-hunting trip to the Oregon Coast for his fifty-fifth birthday in March, at which he smiled a crooked little smile and his gentle blue eyes glistened with tears. In that moment, I believe he finally understood that I would bravely battle the monster with him, faithfully beside him, and would be the one sure thing he could count on. I booked a room at the Coast.

CHAPTER 2

LIVING ON THE EDGE

MARCH IN MONTANA can be a scary time to travel, but we were living on the edge now and didn't really give it much thought. We were going to buy a beach house for Billy's fifty-fifth birthday. We had a plan, and with Jazzy tucked into the backseat on a dreary, snow-covered day in March, we set out. A few hours later we slipped into the Rocky Mountains and began winding up and over Roger's Pass, slowly blazing a trail through a blanket of fresh and slippery snow covering the narrow highway. Climbing *up* the pass allowed us to gratefully hug the rugged wall of rock glaring through Billy's passenger window while cumbersome logging trucks, bogged down with loads of freshly cut pine, squeezed by on the opposite side. I gripped the wheel and held my breath each time they were forced to ramble precariously close to the soft shoulder separating their eighteen wheels from the steep ravine far below. Gigantic snowflakes swirled madly and had gathered into mounds on the hood when we finally inched our way back down the pass and into the tiny mountain town of Lincoln. My first attempt at wild abandon had left my limbs with an exhilarated tingle.

Lincoln, Montana had always been the first of several routine pit stops on our usual route to the beach, and after fueling up we headed for the familiar convenience store to fill our travel mugs with fresh hot coffee. We shook the fluffy flakes from our hair as we entered the brightly lit store and found it bustling with chattering travelers. We overheard several of them expressing concern about continuing westbound due to even heavier snowfall and little or no visibility. Pondering our options reminded us of the reason travel through the vast state of Montana during the months of winter and spring is so unpredictable and dangerous. Knowing our daughter, Autumn, was awaiting our arrival in Missoula just eighty miles southwest of Lincoln, I dialed her number on my cell phone hoping she could give us a report of the weather there. Greeting us cheerfully, she assured us that although the skies in Missoula were overcast, no snow had fallen since the previous evening, leaving us hopeful that the storm cell passing through Lincoln would likely relent if we pressed on westward through the worst of it. We nodded in agreement, threw caution to the wind and forced the tires back onto the slick, snow-covered highway. The next hour was as treacherous as travel in Montana can be, but just as I turned on the wipers once more to clear the windshield, the snow abruptly stopped and the highway was suddenly clear and dry. Thankful for the reprieve, I turned up the music and filled the car with the raspy voice of Billy's favorite Neil Young album for the final forty miles to Missoula.

The alignment of Autumn's schedule with ours was one of the first of many strategically placed gifts The Giver had begun to reveal. Autumn had been completely inundated during the past four years with a rigorous nursing school schedule that she completed only weeks before. She'd also just passed her state nursing exam and because she had not yet begun the arduous process of job hunting, was more than willing to help us choose the setting for our new season at the beach. Her peaceful presence would most certainly wrangle my anxiety into a quiet corner and keep my nervous feet planted firmly in the moment. The instant she wrapped her tiny arms around me I became charged with optimism.

The heavy Rocky Mountain cloud blanketing Missoula early the next morning felt nearly close enough to touch, and the smell of pine through the dense air of spring cleared my lungs of the remaining stagnant bits left behind by winter. We stuffed Autumn's cheery polka-dotted duffle bag into the trunk and settled in to bravely face the mountain passes of Idaho, but not before we made our next routine stop at the Fifty Thousand Dollar Bar in Haugen, Montana.

Nestled even deeper into the magnificent Rocky Mountains, this quaint and popular stop for tourists proudly displays a collection of fifty thousand silver dollars in the barroom where people from all over the world have had their names inscribed next to their inlaid silver dollars in the bar top and on the walls. This had always been one of Autumn's favorite stops during our family trips over the years, and once she had her fill of browsing nostalgically through the gift shop collecting souvenirs and trinkets for friends, we stepped back outside, filled our lungs with another dose of crisp mountain air, fastened our seat belts and prepared for the wintry mountain passes beckoning us into their lair.

By mid-afternoon we had crossed the Montana border into Idaho at the slushy summit of Lookout Pass and wound back down between tunnels of snow left behind by a plow's blade. It wasn't long before we crested the summit of Fourth of July Pass, slipped past the shimmering indigo surface of Lake Coeur d'Alene, and bumped our way through the busy traffic of Spokane. We had always fueled up in Ritzville, and it seemed even more desolate in March than it did during our trips in the heat of summer. We quickly filled our bellies with fast food, gave Jazzy a much-needed walk, and eagerly made our way onto the exit toward The Dalles, Oregon, where Billy's mom was also waiting to join us.

It was early evening when we finally turned onto the shady street lined with hundred-year-old trees to find her sitting patiently on the crooked front steps of her aged Victorian home. Grandma Joyce did not allow Billy's diagnosis to take root in her quiet world of solitude and refused to acknowledge symptoms apparent to even the least-trained eye. She hugged each of us in normal fashion, dragged her frayed luggage over the tattered turf covered steps and smashed it into the backseat, leaving just enough room for her tiny frame to squeeze in next to it.

Joyce exists in a cocoon of self-preservation decorated with recycled things and mystical tools required to slant reality into a spiritual haven. The gentle man she had shared her later years with had slowly faded into heaven's abyss within the prior decade, and only the ordinary construed into angelic signs have allowed her the reserve of passion necessary to integrate with the constantly moving world around her. Following the divorce, the miles had become a difficult obstacle for Joyce when Billy, and his younger brother, Rick, chose to live with their father in Montana. Including her in our new season of memory gathering became part of the plan.

I had often heard about spring storms on the coast, but had never experienced the intensity of one. I welcomed the wild abandon, and as we pulled into the hotel parking lot of the Looking Glass Inn in Lincoln City, the wipers were on high speed and not keeping up with the deluge. By the time we made several trips up to our second floor hotel room through the wind and pounding rain, all of us and everything we brought needed a bit of time to dry out by the fireplace before we left for dinner.

Mo's Restaurant, famous for their clam chowder, was directly across the street from the hotel, and because Mo's had been a traditional dining spot for us, we were more than willing to brave the storm once again.

Mo's sits at the very edge of Siletz Bay, and from a window seat, diners find themselves captivated by a variety of beachy entertainment. Sea lions can be seen sunning themselves on the opposite side of the bay, seagulls caw and battle on the shore, and beach fires smoldering near the water's edge fill the air with an intoxicating blend of campfire smoke and salty sand. The roaring gateway at the entrance of the bay sucks it empty when the tide retreats and fills it back up when the tide rolls in, forcing waves to crash past the pier and high onto the rocks just below the windows.

That night, the rain was hammering on the darkened windows

and the bay was shrouded in a blanket of fog that floated mystically through the glow of street lamps. We peered past the rain's fury and into the foggy bay over bowls of buttery chowder and steaming mugs of hot chocolate topped with mounds of whipped cream. Ah, it felt good to be at the beach.

The storm raged on through the night, and Billy raved for weeks afterwards about the sheets of rain backed by hurricane force winds that had threatened to crash through the hotel window while we slept. But the rain gave way to a bit of sunshine the next morning and we quickly prepared for an exhausting day ahead. Our online search had rendered thirty houses between Seaside and Lincoln City for us to compare in two days. So, with the help of a compassionate mortgage broker with a sense of urgency who already had the financing conundrum underway, and Stephanie, the attentive and friendly real estate agent sent to us by our sister-in-law, Molly, we were now ready to make it happen.

Billy's brother, Jamie, and his beautiful wife, Molly, have an energetic family and have always welcomed us with warm hospitality whenever we passed through on our way to the beach. They were once again immediately willing to help in any way possible when we broke the news of Billy's illness. During a season now past they had even graciously invited Levi, our son, to stay with them when he bravely set out on his own at the age of nineteen to begin his undergraduate studies at Portland State University, where he flourished and was eventually accepted into medical school.

Abundant sunshine led the way to Seaside where we had agreed to meet Stephanie, who would light-heartedly guide us to our perfect beach house. Autumn, having the photographic memory we often teased her about, along with a strong eye for detail, was put in charge of tracking each of the homes' pros and cons, and not long into the day, I realized she was also in charge of entertainment. Her quick wit and cheerful mood made the search a joyous adventure, allowing us to once again tuck the purpose of the trip into the recesses of our minds at least for the next few days.

Just a touch of brandy in our morning coffee may have lessened the agony quickly gnawing at our optimism once we had completed our tour of the Seaside homes on our list. We were void of the passion necessary at the time to sterilize, update, completely remodel or landscape what others considered worthy of the outrageous sales prices with which they tagged their precious properties. The day nearly let in that glass-half-empty mood, but with my broken give-a-shit still steering my thoughts, we waved a cheerful goodbye to Seaside and made plans with Stephanie to start out early the next morning in the more familiar community of Lincoln City. Another evening cup of comforting chowder by the bay and time to warm up by the fireplace eased us into a hopeful slumber.

Our spirits were renewed the next morning when another delightful dose of spring sunshine enriched our breakfast of packaged muffins and coffee. Stephanie called early with an ambitious plan to show us as many houses as possible. She had coordinated with homeowners, her other clients, and her family in order to give us priority and the time needed to get the job done. After looking at fifteen houses that first day in Lincoln City, the very first one we saw quickly became everyone's favorite. But because you should never buy the first one you see, we spent another full day comparing all of the others on our list to the first one, and eventually looked at that favorite first one three more times before we all agreed to put in an offer. Finally, over a frosty glass of draft beer and a big old greasy cheeseburger, we signed an offer and began the waiting game and negotiations between buyer and seller, with Stephanie at the helm of the process. It wasn't long before we reached an agreement and we'd bought ourselves a beautiful home on the north end of Lincoln City.

So Stephanie, the gift to us through Molly's connections, and the time we spent following her through some rain, some sunshine, and lots of laughter became a treasured memory in the first pages of our new scrapbook. The surreal beginning of our next season was set into motion.

CHAPTER 3

GIFTS TO BATTLE THE MONSTER

A BELLY FULL of butterflies and steady rain followed me all the way back to Montana where we spent the night in Missoula with Autumn and Ashley, her childhood friend and roommate. A week brimming with Autumn's joyful spirit was topped off with an evening of laughter and catching up with these two delightful young women, which made it difficult to leave them and face the daunting mountain of details now lying before us in order to get our new adventure underway.

The cold wind and snow that greeted us at home the next afternoon quickly evaporated any doubts we had about our hasty decision, and we bravely unloaded the car and got down to business. Tammy, our diligent mortgage broker, assured us of a quick and painless closing on our new mortgage, and suddenly the timing of so many factors became apparent and unexpectedly intertwined. We had recently applied for social security disability and awaited approval. Short-term disability insurance had been reviewing medical records, and Billy's income was dependent upon their agreement that his diagnosis was as serious and permanent as the doctors assured them that it was. The mortgage process hinged upon approval of disability payments, and we needed to place our home on the market and hope for a quick sale for down payment proceeds. Also by that time, it was common knowledge where I worked that my position there would soon be up for grabs, and although my supervisors were understanding and patient, they were wondering when I planned to make my exit.

Shortly after he had begun the regimen of prescribed medications, Billy came back to life so much that at times I wondered why we were turning our lives upside down and self-inflicting so much anxiety upon ourselves. I even considered the possibility that it wasn't the medications that had put the sparkle back into the blue of his eyes and wondered if he may have been misdiagnosed. After all, the tests didn't link a gene to his condition, and it is extremely rare to acquire this disease at such an early age without a genetic component. Statistically, he probably had a better chance of winning the lottery than acquiring Alzheimer's disease at such an early age without a family history of it, which often made me doubt the neurologist's findings and caused me to revert back to the idea that with even more rest and relaxation he would miraculously and permanently become his wild and funny self again.

We *were* given a thorough report of the spinal tap results however, which again indicated the degree of proteins that had taken up residence in Billy's brain, and that fact would continually shock me back into reality whenever the thought of resuming our previous life presented itself.

I recalled the nurse practitioner's words that had bounced around her office that cold morning in January. She had stressed that each patient's battle with this monster is unique, and although the victor is predestined, the battle may rage for a short time or could become a lengthy war of many years. With the renewed sparkle in my Billy's eyes, I prepared for war and planned our future accordingly. We immediately put our house on the market and began showings with a helpful real estate professional who had previously known Billy through connections in the grocery industry. He remembered Billy and was extremely thoughtful from start to closing, which happened within three short months.

Looking back, I could clearly see that Heaven's hand had touched every step of the complicated process, from the heart-wrenching diagnosis to the busy moving day. All of the sleepless, number-crunching nights were unnecessary, and I really just needed to be patient and follow the obvious guidance that left me awestruck at every turn. Our world was bursting at the seams with grace and strength only The Giver could have so generously bestowed upon us each new day. But I remained silently aware that He would also step in as Taker, and it could not have been humanly possible for me alone to have carried the burden of those months without the supernatural forces that lightened the load. Everything seemed to fall so suspiciously, so perfectly into place that even outsiders began to notice, and without a worldly explanation, listening for Heaven's next directive became the focus of my every waking moment. The obscure and neatly-wrapped gifts began to reveal themselves and became tools to battle back the emotional turmoil fueling our roller coaster.

A special one came when Jamie offered to fly from Portland to Montana to help load all of our belongings into a U-Haul and drive that same U-Haul all the way to our new world waiting for us in Lincoln City. He volunteered for this job out of the blue, and explained that we would be the lucky recipients of his need to *burn up* a few days of vacation time. On the heels of that one, came the gift of Levi with a timely break from school and the desire to help with the physical labor required to get us from point A to point B. Levi, like Autumn, also has a cheerful and hard-working spirit and between he and Jamie's jovial demeanors, little room remained for fear and doubt as we made quick work of putting our entire world into the truck on one of the few sunny days we had during that week in June. The unexpected sunshine was yet another vague little gift.

Jamie had lived in our little prairie town of Havre with his father while he earned his college degree, long before Billy and I had moved there, so taking the trip out to help us move allowed him an opportunity to revisit a small piece of his younger years and family history. Coincidentally, this was also the area where both Billy's and my parents and grandparents grew up. A night spent chatting with Billy's mom in The Dalles during our honeymoon also revealed that she and my mother had gone to the same high school in Harlem, Montana many years before. That fascinating bit of history solidified my belief that Billy and I were destined to be together, yet even after traveling the same high school halls for four long years, our paths had not crossed.

Fate finally stepped in nearly a decade later when I worked for a season in the transmission shop that my father had grown into a reputable family business with the help of my mother's intrepid pioneer spirit and the willingness of my brothers to learn the trade.

I swept the floors, cleaned greasy car parts, and ran errands. And one ordinary afternoon in March, after roaming the aisles of the nearby grocery store, reeking of a mechanic's garage, my life was forever altered. I fumbled with my bags in the checkout when his name fell from the lips of our matchmaker and settled deep into my fibers. I stared at her. I wanted her to say his name again. I wanted to drink in the sound of his name again, and I had never even met him.

"Bill Filler," she repeated, "he has the biggest crush on you. He drives a Camaro. He's really nice. Could I give him your number?"

"Um, sure, I guess so." I hesitated, wondering if I had passed by him that afternoon and hadn't even noticed.

I watched as she scratched my number down on a sticky note and stuffed it into her pocket. Bill Filler, Billy they called him—I repeated it over and over again in my head that ordinary afternoon in March. Curiously, I hoped he would call. He did. And that was it. I was an addict and Billy was my drug. Neither my parents nor my brothers were thrilled with his wild side and it took a few break-ups and five proposals before I shunned their reasonable advice and jumped into a new life with my Billy Filler. A wild ride ensued, and during the early years of our marriage, he would often reminisce about the smell of burnt transmission fluid that permeated the aisles he regularly stocked when I wandered by. His smiling eyes would light up and he would give me the special wink and grin that made me fall head over heels in love with him not long after we met.

The warm afternoon quickly faded into a still, crisp evening in Havre, Montana. As the heavy lifting came to an end, I continued with the final details of packing up odds and ends while Billy and Levi accompanied Jamie on a trip down memory lane. A melancholy visit to the local cemetery where their father had been laid to rest a few years before was followed by a nostalgic beer at the Gallery Lounge, a hot spot for college students where Jamie had spent many wild weekends of his own. By the time they returned, chuckling and poking fun at each other as they climbed out of the car, the sun had given way to dusk. With the long drive ahead lurking like another scary beast that needed to be conquered, we headed for our sleeping bags as the warning of a 4:00 a.m. wake-up call from Jamie threatened us into a few hours of sleep.

Right on time, Jamie's stomping echoed through the empty house, and when Levi stepped outside to check on the caravan we had readied for travel, the brightness of the full moon, and the clear Montana sky filled with stars instantly caught his attention. Billy and I shook off the confusion of waking up on a cold, hard floor and answered his call to go out and share in the mystical start to our journey. Jamie was eager and energized and quickly reminded us of the waiting beast we still needed to conquer. His impatient attitude drove us to stuff the last of our belongings into any vacant corner of the truck that we could find. We rubbed our sleepy eyes and each got behind our steering wheels.

It had previously been agreed upon that Jamie would drive the U-Haul, Levi would take the pickup loaded with the camper and tow our treasured fishing boat behind, and Billy would be my co-pilot in his bright orange Grand Prix, which was also loaded floorboards to sunroof. As we pulled away from the curb and our little house became smaller in the rear view mirror, an unexpected sadness twisted in the pit of me. I had gone kicking and screaming when Billy was forced to accept his position in Harlem, Montana. And I had grown a healthy crop of guilt over the past decade when the compromise to live in Havre had caused my Billy to commute a total of eighty-six miles each day over a dangerous stretch of highway through many winter storms. I'd often longed for the day when we could say good-bye to Havre and Harlem forever, but leaving under such sorrow and uncertainty was not what I had hoped for.

I held that moment close for a bit, realizing it would be the last time I'd ever see a full moon shining on our little block of the world, and realizing that I would finally be content to spend all the rest of my days there if only we could conquer Billy's monster. Our dismal future and the long drive suddenly hung heavy, dampening my previously perky mood.

CHAPTER 4

JOURNEY TO THE NEW WORLD

THE SUN ROSE shortly after the trip was underway and stayed with us all the way through the mountain passes of Montana and Idaho, warming the lava beds of southeastern Washington as we slowly worked our way toward Oregon, stopping only for fuel, bathroom breaks and more junk food, as required of any good road trip.

The timing of those stops for fuel and snacks were pertinent once we left the Tri-Cities area of Washington. The long stretch following the Columbia River in the desolate and sparsely populated northern corner of Oregon leaves few opportunities. Levi soon realized that towing his heavy load had used up fuel far quicker than he had anticipated and he soon regretted missing the exit to the gas station many miles back in Pasco. Suddenly, using common sense I rarely gave him credit for, he began to slow his speed in hopes of conserving what little fuel he had left, and the rest of our little caravan soon became concerned as he lagged behind. Cell phones were a lifeline between vehicles and after calls back and forth, we quickly became fearful of the pending possibility that Levi could run out of gas far from anywhere that offered services. We stayed close behind him for several miles and hoped for the best. Another little gift came in the form of a huge, fluorescent green road sign boldly pointing the way to the little town of Rufus just five miles ahead. Rufus is a tiny town set into the rocky hillside overlooking the Columbia River, and the gas station's bright yellow sign was beaming a welcome just beyond the exit. Levi, after puttering on well-conserved fumes, barely coasted up the hill to the first pump. We all climbed out, stretched our legs, breathed a heavy sigh of relief and giggled our way through the little store while our caravan was being refueled.

The adrenaline from our averted crisis left us with a much-needed surge of energy as we gratefully resumed our journey alongside the immense Columbia River. Billy and I turned our attention toward the fearless fishing boats dotting the dark surface, and the tug boats rolling effortlessly through its wide and dangerous waters. While we were captivated by the activity on the river, the sun had lit up the western horizon and dressed the smooth surface of the water in sparkling diamonds that shimmered for miles alongside of us. I filled the car with Billy's music and watched him relax into the seat.

The Dalles came up quickly and a short visit with Grandma left us hoping to reach Jamie's home before the sun fell completely behind the horizon. Suddenly the weather was no longer cooperating and an angry thunder shower poured heavy raindrops onto the winding curves past Cascade Locks, and into Portland's busy evening traffic, making it hard to see past the speeding wipers spraying sheets of rain in all directions. When the worst of the storm finally passed, it left behind billows of ominous dark clouds that floated just above the sunroof, threatening us all the way to Jamie's front door.

Molly's excitement vibrated through the still damp air of the cul-de-sac when we hobbled through the screen door she had braced open with an outstretched arm. The tantalizing smells of her warm kitchen permeated the house and the chaos of family instantly wrapped its welcoming arms around us. The long day blissfully ended with full bellies and weary spirits bathed in red wine. We all slept well that night.

The next day brought a much-needed break from our exhausting journey and we were content to watch our niece play in several local softball games. Jamie and Molly are the proud and busy parents of Ashley, a talented softball player, and her younger sister, Maddy, a quick-witted teenager who plays a mean game of basketball. Weekends with family are important to them, and Jamie was thrilled to be home in time to watch Ashley play in an important and exciting game.

Billy and I soaked up Levi's light-hearted spirit from the sidelines on that cool, dew-covered morning. The smell of glistening pine trees and damp bark dust beneath colorful flower gardens filled the air. The sun did its best to warm us while low clouds continued to meander through its path. I closed my eyes and breathed in deeply, recalling why I loved this part of the world. Billy had become completely enthralled in the man-to-man time he shared with Levi, and my heart nearly burst with pride from the attention my son gave his father and the resulting joy that perked up Billy's weary face. I watched in peaceful admiration, and the by-product of fatigue that followed my decision to uproot our entire world slowly evaporated with the morning dew. Spending the entire day cheering for Ashley's team in the sunshine and fresh air left us recharged and ready to face the remainder of our journey and the hard work of unloading the overstuffed U-Haul truck when we claimed our new home the next afternoon.

Molly's cheerful spirit broke the morning's stillness and engulfed the kitchen, along with the aroma of freshly brewed coffee and hearty sizzling breakfast treats as we made our way downstairs. The guys filled their plates and teased each other about who had worked the hardest and had the sorest muscles due to all of the hard moving they had previously endured. I giggled softly and passed Billy the first cup of coffee Molly sweetly handed me. I knew right away that she would be a helpful friend should I need one and my trust in her kind and willing spirit was immediate. Her warm, filling breakfast readied us for the long day ahead, and we barely finished the last bite when Jamie once again impatiently pressured us into getting back behind the wheel.

Our caravan wove slowly through the heavy morning traffic and finally onto the less traveled highway leading to the beach. Small farms draped with rambling vineyards framed the emerald Willamette Valley, glowing and bathed in morning sunshine. And as if the gleaming valley weren't spectacular enough, we soon slipped into the VanDuzer Corridor, a seemingly endless tunnel of sky-piercing Oregon pines tethered to the loamy soil by shallow roots with fern-laden foliage tangled tightly around their trunks. The brilliance of unusual spring sunshine burst through the windshield between bouncing branches, nearly blinding me as we rolled through the winding curves of the corridor, and although I was excited to see our new home again, I was not eager for the serenity of our journey to end.

But right on schedule, we rumbled into our new neighborhood, shattering the peacefulness I would soon come to realize was a consistent amenity of our picture perfect subdivision. The dense and undeveloped forest located directly across the street lent itself as a pleasant distraction when we took breaks from the unloading of heavy boxes and furniture, and the time-consuming task of finding a place for household goods that quickly clogged every inch of floor space. The damp heat of the afternoon snuffed out the final flame of energy we all had that morning just as the last of the boxes had been shuffled into the remaining corners of the garage.

Shortly after Levi and Jamie had returned the obtrusive U-Haul truck and devoured several slices of steaming pizza, Billy and I found them snoring next to each other on air mattresses thrown near the fireplace in the living room. The sight of them soundly sleeping in the same clothes they had worked so hard in through the heat and humidity all day, left me with a grateful grin. I quickly locked up and showed Billy to our freshly made bed, already set up in our new bedroom at the beach.

CHAPTER 5

BUILDING OUR BUBBLE

ALTHOUGH WE AWOKE the next morning to heavy gray skies and a slow drizzle of rain, that Monday in June would mark the beginning of a very significant summer and a season in what would become our *bubble at the beach*, the surreal new world that would remain our refuge for as long as The Giver would allow.

Jamie was ready to rejoin his family and the duties of his own life after his generous donation of time, and Levi willingly drove him back to Portland that morning with the promise of returning a few days later after visiting a special friend there. The quiet was deafening once they had gone and I quickly busied myself with removing the chaos that surrounded us.

Billy was eager to help and it was easy at that time to find chores that he had the ability to complete without much assistance. He spent many hours in the coolness of the garage breaking down the boxes I continued to empty, and he made an impressive attempt at organizing the workbench that had been buried beneath random buckets, tools, and plastic totes.

Once I had unpacked most of the boxes, I was surprised at how quickly and easily all of our belongings fell into place, as if everything already had a designated home, and with very little effort I simply put things *away*. I took frequent breaks to check on Billy and drew him outside often to stand in the mist and listen to the rumble of the Pacific Ocean just beyond the forest. We mostly stood in silence. The evolvement into the quiet man my Billy had become was a stark contrast to his previous outspoken and social personality. I found myself continually intrigued by the apathy that quickly replaced the fiery spirit he embodied not so very long ago. He inhaled deeply. The cool breeze gently caressed our warm skin and washed a calming peace over us, momentarily relieving the apprehension we never discussed.

Great progress was made throughout the afternoon, and by the time evening crept in, our bubble had begun to feel like home. I sat a steaming bowl of tomato soup and a plate of grilled cheese sandwiches in front of Billy when he finally pulled a stool up to the counter, and while the soup did its best to comfort us, we began to wish we still had the well-worn, leaky hot tub sitting empty on our deck back in Montana. Billy had always enjoyed relaxing in the warm, swirling water after throwing freight throughout the day in the deep cold of winter. A good soak after dinner that night would have been a perfect ending to our productive day. Knowing a new tub for our backyard was high on our summer project list made it easier to settle for a long steamy shower before snuggling in for the night.

Although we awoke once more to a steady drizzle of rain, we hugged our mugs of warm coffee under the protection of the covered porch and nodded in agreement that come rain or shine, we would find a shortcut to the beach through the dripping forest that beckoned us from beneath its blanket of morning fog. A hearty breakfast and the rain gear we'd purchased during our house hunting trip in March prepared us for the adventure at hand. Once Jazzy had been wrangled into her yellow rain slicker, we set out to explore our new world.

The forest was actually a subdivision in progress that had apparently been abandoned after the real estate market crash of 2008, and we sheepishly grinned at each other when we slipped through the wide metal gate bearing a large "No Trespassing" sign boldly cautioning us in bright red letters. We crested the hill of a professionally paved, yet untraveled city street and found ourselves whispering in the eerie silence. Creeping gingerly over the damp pavement, we paused to study the overgrown weeds crowding sidewalks and partially installed utility lines. It could have easily been a scene from a science fiction film where the entire community was snatched up by aliens. A brisk wind caused the tall pines, still dripping with rain and tipped with fog, to wave wildly far above us, and a crow suddenly appeared and cawed what seemed to be warnings. Our eyes darted nervously from one side of the vacant street to the other with Jazzy obliviously leading the way, pulling at the end of her leash and stopping only to violently shake her entire body as if to reinstate her hatred of the slicker we had fastened around her chubby underbelly. We rounded the bend into a lonely would-be cul-de-sac and spotted a beaten down path leading into the forest still hidden from view. Once we had pushed our way through the tangles of overgrown blackberry bushes and ferns, the forest path opened up into a wide shady tunnel beneath ancient towering pines.

Low, leafless branches covered in bright green moss reached eerily down toward the damp blanket of decomposing leaves that we had intruded upon, and our cumbersome rain boots echoed through the silence as we plodded along.

Every now and then our clumsy boots would nearly crush a fat banana slug, its pale yellow exterior and unnaturally long slimy body blending into the musty mix. I kept a vigilant eye for a lone coyote or mountain lion rumored to roam through the underbrush, while Billy's face glowed with enchantment at the historic beauty encircling us.

He bent down to pick up a broken branch, examined it for use as a walking stick, and after tapping it and putting it to good use for a few yards, he reached down and picked up another. Before long he had several sticks under his arm and informed me of his intention to haul all of them home and create a supply of walking sticks for future visitors to enjoy. My heart skipped a beat with the hope that my Billy had already discovered a productive way to fill his abundant free time.

Another metal gate bearing a bold "No Trespassing" sign greeted us at the end of the path, warning anyone entering from that side of the forest. We slipped around the corner of the gate and stowed the cache of sticks we had gathered near the path's edge with a plan to retrieve them on our way back through the forest after visiting the beach. The air was heavy with salt and earth, and we tramped hand-in-hand down a muddy graveled road lined with more huge ferns popping through thick tangles of thorny blackberry bushes. A creek babbling loudly over fallen logs spilled into a mossy pond, catching our attention and interrupting our musings of several large homes tucked discreetly amongst the tall pines barely rooted into the damp and steep hillside. We were still chatting about the glistening emerald head of a duck we had seen fluffing his feathers at the edge of the pond when we rounded the final bend and felt a salty mist prickle our cheeks.

The state park that led to the surf's edge was suddenly in our sights and we realized the entire walk took only twenty minutes including time to gather walking sticks. The thrill of finding the shortcut we had hoped for on our first day out, and not getting eaten by a rogue wild animal in the process, put a spring in our step and we nearly skipped the rest of the way to the park over slippery beach stones that stood between us and the crashing waves.

The weather was less than desirable for beach walks and miles of uninhabited sand stretched out far on each side of us. Cascade Head, a well-known headland sat regally in the center of the pounding surf to the right, and heavy clouds of misty gray mingled with the watery horizon stretched out far to the left.

The Oregon Coast is an indescribable sight to behold regardless of how the weather transforms it and we stood silent in the prickly breeze, drinking in the delicious salty air before we turned for our trek back home.

We plodded back over the muddy road and met the first gate just a few minutes later, loaded our arms with the harvest of sticks and clambered back into the forest.

Levi was true to his word and returned a few days later, bringing not only his lighthearted and helpful spirit with him, but also a very pretty friend who helped make the precious little time remaining of his visit even more memorable. We put life's duties on hold and spent the weekend partaking in local tourist attractions which included a summer kite festival on the windy beach, sauntering through the dampness of an outdoor farmers market, stuffing our bellies with fresh pastries from a local bakery, and dining on chowder from a window seat at a beachfront restaurant. Time passed far too quickly and after sharing with them the tranquility we'd found in our shortcut to the beach, we spent our final evening together roasting hot dogs and marshmallows over a cozy fire in the chiminea under another magical, star-filled sky in our brand new bubble.

Unfortunately, I was reminded of the fragility of our bubble's shell that evening shortly after tucking Billy into bed. Levi and I had irresponsibly lost track of how often his wine glass had been refilled, and by the time we left coals smoldering in the chiminea and went inside, the wine's effects had taken hold of his already impaired speech and gait. It took no coercing to get him into bed and I stayed up with Levi and checked on him often. He had been soundly sleeping for an hour or so when I heard him stirring in the darkened room. I rushed in to find him still lying in bed, appearing to be fully awake but reaching his arms straight out and wriggling his fingers as if he were beckoning someone to his bedside. He began muttering incoherently to someone or something he seemed convinced was right there in the room with him. I tiptoed to his side, bent down near his face and whispered,

"I'm right here, Billy."

His blank stare focused on mine for just a moment before he began to scramble from beneath the covers, attempting to get out of bed. I assumed he needed to use the bathroom and locked our elbows together as he wobbled up onto shaky legs. I guided him to the bathroom where I turned on a light, hoping the brightness would snap him out of the trance currently controlling his reality. I breathed a sigh of relief when he used the bathroom without assistance, and it appeared that he saw *me* as I turned him back toward the bedroom and our eyes met. That relief retreated when he suddenly broke the grasp I had on his elbow, stretched both arms out to the side as far as he possibly could, put his chin up high, and with clarity I hadn't heard in months, said emphatically,

"I have no idea where I just was, but I want to go back there. All I know is that I do *not* want to be *here*!"

He began to cry, dropped his hands and shoulders in exhaustion, took my hand and allowed me to lead him back to his side of the bed. I covered his chilled body with the warm blankets, kissed him softly, whispered "I love you, Billy," and studied him closely as he drifted back to sleep.

I was bewildered, and replayed what had just happened over and over again in my mind. Was it a reaction to the combination of alcohol and medication? Had his heart stopped? Had he visited heaven for a moment? In exasperation I did my best to explain to Levi what I had witnessed, and we were eager to interrogate him when he awoke the next morning. But an explanation would elude us. Billy puttered around the kitchen as if nothing strange at all had happened, and when we gently prodded for details, he could not recall a single second of the strange episode. We would be left to wonder.

CHAPTER 6

SUNSHINE AND STICKS

IN AN ATTEMPT to capture the serenity befitting life at the beach, I spent the next few rainy days after Levi's departure with laborious efforts at decorating, and when coveted rays of sunshine finally began to pour through the blinds and light up the entire house, it quickly became much less interesting. Although a few strategically integrated home décor items acquired from several local tourist shops had added a bit of ambiance into my haphazard attempt at interior design, I eventually gave myself permission to shrug my shoulders in temporary approval and wandered out to the garage to check on Billy.

I found him fervently stripping the bark from the moss-covered sticks we'd gathered and instantly I forgot about the decorating and gave in to my desire to spend the afternoon with him outdoors. With the warmth of the welcome sunshine came the familiar musty scent of the damp earth wafting through the coolness of the shaded garage. I sneaked up behind him with hopes of startling him out of deep concentration and evoking a shocked gasp and the laughter that was sure to follow whenever we inflicted that cruel behavior upon each other. He did not disappoint me and jerked around with his pocket knife in hand, letting out the expected gasp followed by an annoyed chuckle. After realizing it was only me, he immediately began an excited, but stumbling attempt at describing the progress he had made on his first few walking sticks.

One of the first signs of the monster's presence was Billy's inability to recall appropriate words before a thought was lost altogether. I often struggled with the urge to complete sentences for him, hoping to alleviate the frustration I assumed he must have felt, yet rarely expressed. But this time I refrained from guessing and patiently allowed him the time he needed to find the right words on his own. Once he understood my sincere interest in what he was trying to tell me, he held the partially stripped stick out for me to admire and slowly began pointing out the natural carvings deep in the wood. Taking his time, and speaking with slow clarity, he told me that he felt the stick held a story that would be revealed as he stripped the outer layer of bark away and exposed the hidden markings beneath. My spirit sank a little, for few of those blessed to be a part of my Billy's world had made an effort to strip away his outer layer of protective bark and discover the scarred and gentle man shielded beneath.

The solace he had found in his new niche was heartwarming and I was quick to encourage him with praise and approval. The lyrics of his favorite Neil Young album floated gently on the cool afternoon breeze, and we held each other long, there amongst the bark shavings.

After I'd spent some time surveying the freshly organized garage, Billy became aware of my intention to remain in his space and suggested that we investigate the tangled pile of broken tree limbs stacked just beyond the gate to the abandoned subdivision. Showing clear enthusiasm for his new hobby became my focus and I joined in on the task of collecting sticks. And while he gathered straight strong ones to build his inventory, I carefully chose the smaller ones with sprawling wispy limbs still attached at their tops. Most of them had natural burgundy-colored bark and we later learned that they were an abundant weed regularly demolished in an attempt to eradicate them altogether. We thought they were perfect and proudly dragged them home with plans to protect their natural beauty under a coat or two of varnish before turning them into works of art. Billy had a good

29

start on his walking sticks, but I had other ideas for my selection of wispy limbs.

When we left our home in Montana, much of our well-worn furniture was left behind, requiring us to replace it when we moved in. A guest bed was one of the first new items we acquired and because our budget was well-planned-out and an expensive headboard was not considered a necessity, my creative side sparked into action and I arranged several branches with the wispy limbs still attached into a row on the sunny driveway, picturing them as a whimsical replacement. We had purchased several cans of amber-colored shellac for finishing the walking sticks and I sneaked into the garage to borrow a can for my project too. Billy shot me a sly grin, but was quick to share and I set out to shine up my branches before I attached them to a few of the larger, straighter sticks he had also reluctantly allowed me to borrow from his stash.

I had been sitting on the hard concrete of the driveway, meticulously varnishing each sprig of each branch, when the two young neighbor girls popped out from behind the fence, giggling and chasing Jazzy around the front yard. Their playful laughter echoed through the air and immediately made the already bright sun appear even brighter. They were full of questions about what I was creating while Jazzy tugged at their sleeves and chased the ball they repeatedly threw down the sidewalk. I was describing what my branches were being transformed into, when their sun-kissed faces and energetic spirits flooded my mind with memories of the days when Levi and Autumn bounced around me every day. Their joyful presence was welcome, and after convincing their father that they had not intruded, they stayed for a while and allowed me the pleasure of absorbing a bit of their bountiful energy.

Just as the girls' mother stepped outside to call them in for dinner, an instant damp breeze replaced the warmth of the sun as it slipped behind the forest. By that time I had fashioned my sticks into the headboard I had somewhat envisioned, and after Billy helped me carry it carefully into the guest room, we fastened it proudly behind the bed. I adorned it even further that evening with twinkle lights, and it seemed to bring a bit of the night sky indoors with us. I found the whimsy of my new creation comforting and had big plans to give purpose to many more of the sticks Billy continued to painstakingly strip and varnish.

CHAPTER 7

BUGS AND BARK

WITH THE WARMER weather came the eagerness to prepare the back yard for the hot tub we hoped to have installed before the steady rains of fall arrived. The project began with the removal of an impractical layer of landscape bark adorning the entire yard, and after several walks to explore our new neighborhood, it soon became apparent that this bark was used in abundance. The contractor obviously intended to prevent erosion in the most economical and low-maintenance way possible. To our dismay, a variety of creeping insects and an abundance of incredibly speedy spiders had put down roots beneath the bark, forcing us to retreat to the safety of the porch. Due to my unfounded, yet uncontrollable fear of the speedy eight-legged creatures, replacing the bark with soft green grass on one side and concrete for our tub on the other became necessary and immediate. We put stick hunting trips and visits to the beach on hold and spent our days filling our shiny new wheelbarrow with bark from the back yard, maneuvering it cautiously down the steep hill of even deeper bark in the front yard, and across the street to the growing pile that had been started by several homeowners before us.

Randy and Jenn, our neighbors on one side, had obviously made generous donations to the neighborhood pile, as their yard was already void of the pesky bark. A functioning patio and a soft green glow from their freshly-seeded lawn had begun to take its place. A spark of envy when we pulled up next to our own bark-laden yard on moving day was quickly replaced with gratitude when we each spotted the newly constructed fence that now separated Randy's freshly renovated yard from ours.

We had been warned by Stephanie after making the offer on our house that installing the fence would be our responsibility in order to obscure the unsightly camper we intended to park permanently between our homes. Jamie was especially relieved as he had not only committed himself to helping with the move and the long drive from Montana to Oregon, but had also generously offered to help build the required fence. Billy and I immediately took Jamie's wise advice and introduced ourselves with an offer to share in the expense of fencing materials. Without hesitation Randy and Jenn graciously accepted our offer and became an instant resource whenever we needed answers about landscaping or our new community.

Before resuming the tedious task of bark removal, we began each new day silently lingering with a cozy mug of fragrant coffee on the front step, captivated by the morning light bouncing from one bobbing pine bough to another and momentarily transforming the forest into a mesmerizing display of sparkling dewdrops. Every now and then a family of deer sauntered by, stopping for a moment to give us a puzzled look, or a brightly colored hummingbird whizzed by for a quick drink of nectar from a brightly colored blossom.

The silence was often broken when a friendly neighbor rounded the bend with their puppies prancing beside them, greeting us as they passed by. At the sight of another puppy, Jazzy would leap into action from her warm spot on the concrete and bound into the street, bringing about instant chaos. Some would take the time to say hello to Jazzy and introduce their puppy, but others were understandably unappreciative of our lack of manners in letting Jazzy roam free, and though we were slow learners in the beginning, we finally relented and began using the leash *most* mornings.

It was our lack of puppy etiquette that prompted our neighbor on the other side to stop by and introduce himself during one of our morning coffee breaks. Ryan, a Fish and Wildlife officer, gently warned us that Jazzy could be an easy target of a lone coyote or even a turkey vulture without the tether of her leash. Several of the neighborhood walkers had shared stories of mountain lion and bear sightings in the forest too, so I took the opportunity to ask Ryan if the fear of a mountain lion attack during our stick hunting trips in the forest was realistic. He attempted to make me feel less fearful of what was lurking behind the thick underbrush during our walks.

Meanwhile, Billy brought his attention to the boat sitting untouched in the garage. Fishing during the summer months in Montana was a passion of Billy's and although he could no longer be the captain of the boat he was so proud of, he was eager to have it licensed and ready for fishing and crabbing in Oregon. Ryan was quick to give us all of the resources and contacts necessary, and explained them in detail as he handed me his business card. I studied the card while they looked over the boat and quietly chuckled to myself when I noticed that our *new* neighbor and our hardworking young neighbor we were so fond of back in Montana, not only had the same first name, but also the same last name minus one letter. That uncanny coincidence, and our instant trust in Ryan, left me feeling even more safely nestled into our quiet corner of this new world. A divine hand was surely guiding us and leaving spirit-catching signs of His constant presence in the most unusual of places. A peaceful smile snuck up on me as the *new* Ryan drove away.

The morning sun quickly inched higher into the sky and we turned our attention back to the last of the bark standing between us and the beautiful green grass we had envisioned. For the next few hours, I scraped the remaining embedded bark into piles, and Billy scooped it into the wheelbarrow and repeatedly added it to the growing pile across the street. When he didn't return promptly from one of his trips to the bark pile, I peeked over the fence to check on him and found that he had stopped to chat with Jim, a gentleman who had introduced himself while walking his dogs shortly after we moved in. Billy was quick to share his Alzheimer's diagnosis with Jim, and I was moved by Jim's compassionate patience whenever Billy's attempt at idle small talk was riddled with misplaced words and incoherent sentences. Jim would nod and carry on with the conversation as if everything Billy had uttered made perfect sense, and that seemed to leave Billy a little more confident that he was holding his own against the monster.

When he finally returned with the empty wheelbarrow, he was excited to tell me that Jim had invited us to stop by for strawberry shortcake that his wife had made, and they were expecting us within half an hour. We were both happy to take a break, and after changing our clothes and washing off the layer of dirt covering our hands and faces, we walked the short distance to Jim's house and found him already preparing the patio table with glasses of icy lemonade and bowls of shortcake topped with fresh strawberries and whipped cream. We were soon joined by Jim's wife who made us feel instantly at ease and for a while we escaped within the sweetness of the shortcake and friendly conversation.

Jim was also an avid fisherman and we relaxed into his stories of salmon fishing in the deep and dangerous waters of the powerful Pacific. But before long the late afternoon breeze turned much cooler and we waved goodbye with the promise of a fishing adventure together in the near future.

With a chilly fog wafting through the neighborhood and shortcake filling our bellies, the desire to tackle the remaining piles of bark when we returned home had all but disappeared, so we finished up the day with a long hot shower and a plan for an early start the next morning.

CHAPTER **8**

FOR THE LOVE OF JAZZY

OUR VISION OF velvety green grass was slowly becoming a reality. We removed the last of the bark the next morning and began replacing it with loads of topsoil from a pyramid of dark earthy dirt that had been piled up next to the mounds of discarded bark. Throughout the next week, Billy brought load after load while I raked and leveled in preparation for seed. Dust and sweat covered his handsome face. Exhausted, he finally plopped down on the back step, and with a heavy sigh emphatically declared the yard ready to plant. I surveyed the topsoil I had carefully leveled, checked for depth and clumps, and after taking note of the fatigue so obviously consuming my Billy, I heartily agreed with him. He leaned back into the sun while I generously sprinkled the tiny little seeds all over the freshly raked topsoil, gave it an even sprinkling with the garden hose and sat down next to him with a well-deserved bottle of icy cold beer. We proudly admired our accomplishment and prayed for a week of germinating sunshine.

Our prayers for days of uninterrupted sunshine were answered and brought with them a perfect opportunity for Jamie, Molly, and the girls to visit for a weekend of fun in the sun at the beach while the seeds of our new lawn took root. We were excited to share our steadily evolving bubble with family and happy that they were also bringing Milo, their Yorkshire terrier, to romp with Jazzy. Busy with the yard, we had not been giving Jazzy the attention to which she'd been accustomed and a good run on the beach with Milo would give her some much-needed exercise and companionship. Jazzy had realized the freedom of running on the beach during our first few sunny visits there and entertained us frequently afterwards with the *pug shuffle* her breed is known for. Tucking her tail between her legs and keeping her back end low to the ground, she ran at break-neck speed making huge figure eights in the sand, stopping only to make a happy grunt and start all over again.

They arrived early, and shortly after duffle bags, blankets, pillows, and snacks had spilled out of the bed of their pickup and were scattered haphazardly throughout the house, we scrambled back into the pickup. Squished between my nieces and buried under bouncing puppies and excited chatter, Billy and I endured the short mile to the beach access at Roads End.

Rarely does the wind at the beach relent during the summer months and we intended to take full advantage of the perfect weather. We loaded our arms with beach blankets and sand toys, stumbled over mounds of slippery stones, climbed over massive redwood logs left behind by winter's high surf, and traipsed through the warm sand in search of the perfect spot to spread out our blankets and spend the entire day soaking up the sun.

We were soon stretched out on blankets, lulled by the roar of the ocean and ingesting the salty air and sunshine. The intrigue of Cascade Head began to beckon, and with very little coaxing, the girls and the puppies were ready to join in for a nice long walk to the tide pools at the far end of the beach. We wrapped the straps of Billy's freshly made walking sticks around our wrists and started out for an hour or two of beachcombing. Jazzy did not disappoint us, showing her enthusiasm with several pug shuffles while repeatedly fetching empty mussel shells strewn abundantly over the sand. Milo watched with a confused cock of his head between his own absurd displays of protectiveness when other dogs passed by.

Milo is obviously not aware of his lack of height and stature when

his instincts take over, and he charges wildly at the many large re-
trievers chasing balls thrown into the surf by their owners. Luckily,
their confusion at his silly display, accompanied by the hard jerk at
the end of his leash, usually deferred a confrontation. After momentarily staring at him in bewilderment, the larger dogs would snatch
up their balls and nonchalantly prance away, leaving Milo feeling a
smidge taller and even more confident that it was his tough demeanor
causing them to retreat.

Captivated for some time by the song of the surf, and the abundance of sea life exposed by the low tide once we had reached
Cascade Head, we hadn't been aware of the sun's growing intensity,
and Jazzy and Milo soon lost their playfulness and were in need of a
cool drink of water. With our pockets bulging with beach treasures,
we began a brisk walk back to our blankets where the puppies could
lap up cool water and rest in the damp sand.

We basked throughout the afternoon, feasted on turkey sandwiches and watched the girls build sandcastles before we began to
shake out the blankets and brush the sand from toys and puppies.
But just as we had turned to go, we became mesmerized by several
kite surfers that had appeared directly in front of us. Covered head to
toe in the safety of a wet suit and tethered to their boards by a giant
kite billowing in the wind far above them, they rode the surf out to a
frightening distance and caught a rolling wave with their boards just
as their brightly colored kites sent them flying into the air far above
the icy water.

Gliding effortlessly back to the surf's edge and bucking the roaring waves back out, they continued their dance on the glistening water and we remained their captivated audience. We were blissfully
unaware that the brilliant gold of the warm afternoon sun had turned
to a shimmering orange and had begun its evening descent. The instant chilly breeze signaled us to pack up before the glowing orange
ball on the horizon completely disappeared behind the indigo water
far in the distance.

Jamie, Molly, and the girls filled the entire house with chaos and laughter throughout the weekend. But once the chaos had been stuffed back into their pickup and we waved goodbye as they slipped around the bend, the silence left in their wake was once again unwelcome and deafening. In my previous life, I had always appreciated the peace found through periods of silence during the day, but the lack of comfort I now found in the quiet was disconcerting and immediately opened the door to frightening visions of Billy's inevitable descent into ultimate dependency, and the growing uncertainty of my ability to honor him with the patience and fortitude he deserved. In an effort to keep the intrusive reminders at bay, I found myself filling every silent moment with projects, prayers, and medicinal doses of red wine.

We lingered with our coffee on the sun-drenched front step longer than we usually did after they had gone that morning, and even Jazzy felt much less energetic. To our surprise, she didn't even acknowledge the morning walkers with a round of protective barks and growls as they strolled by right in front of her. The sun became increasingly warmer. We noticed she began to pant loudly at our feet, her stomach contracting deeply in and slowly back out. Assuming she was too warm, we tried to coax her into the shade, but she would not budge and her belly continued to lurch painfully in and out. It was soon apparent that something was terribly wrong and we frantically began to search for a local vet that would see her on short notice. The first one we called instructed us to bring her right in, and by the time we arrived at the office, Jazzy was completely lethargic and extremely cold. The doctor took her drooping body from my arms and asked us to return in a few hours after she had time to examine Jazzy and test a sample of blood.

Her concerned expression left us even more anxious and we fought back tears at the fear of losing Jazzy so unexpectedly. Billy was shaking, and we waited helplessly. I prayed that the doctor could bring us back the playful companion that we had romped on the beach with just the day before.

I recalled the shivering little, long-legged puppy Billy brought home from work with him that frigid November evening three years ago. Billy and Jazzy became inseparable during the months they spent home alone together back in Montana, and her playfulness and funny personality kept him busy and upbeat during weeks of winter's bitter cold while I was away at work. I knew losing Jazzy would be very difficult for Billy, and my silent prayers continued throughout the next hours that seemed to drag on forever.

My cell phone finally rang and the doctor urged us to take Jazzy to a specialist in Beaverton as her blood results revealed possible liver failure. After a moment of initial shock, we understood the seriousness of the situation and immediately set out on the two hour drive to Beaverton. We reached the office just as they were ready to close for the day and even though Jazzy was much warmer by then and able to stand on her own, the doctor suggested we leave her overnight for observation. Gratefully leaving her in his qualified hands, we agreed to call for an update the next morning. Jamie and Molly welcomed us in for the night, and although we were happy to hear that Milo showed no signs of illness after spending the weekend with Jazzy, we were even more confused at what could have caused her to become so very sick so quickly.

Jazzy had made a miraculous recovery by the time we called the next morning, but the doctor explained that her recovery was most likely due to the electrolyte injection she received by the vet in Lincoln City. Her liver enzymes were still extremely high and he warned us that her health could deteriorate quickly again without further tests and proper treatment. With the doctor's approval we took Jazzy home, promising to keep a watchful eye.

Over the next few weeks Jazzy slowly regained her spunkiness, and showed no further signs of illness. When we finally felt it was safe to take her back to the beach, we were much wiser and offered her plenty of fresh water. Our Jazzy had survived to run many more pug shuffles through the salty sand.

CHAPTER 9

A BREATH OF FRESH AIR

JULY BROUGHT WITH it patches of bright green popping up sporadically throughout the damp earth on which we had toiled so hard. The remainder of the yard seemed forlorn and forgotten since we'd left it untouched after the bark eradication, but I had been quietly contemplating its transformation and the addition of the hot tub we were planning to pick out with Autumn's help during her upcoming visit.

Autumn had been diligently applying for nursing jobs once she had her hard-earned license in hand; but with a resumé void of experience, quickly became discouraged by constant rejections from local medical facilities and hospitals. An uplifting weekend visit to our bubble became a temporary remedy. The weather was gray and drizzly from the moment she stepped off the plane in Portland until we dropped her off again a few days later. But the mist only added to the serenity of the beach, and shortly after we deposited her luggage into the guest room, we donned our rain jackets and headed down to the colorful tide pools.

Reminiscent of the imaginative and bright-eyed little girl she was just a blink ago, tears wriggled past my lids as I watched her bounce barefooted over the sand with her snazzy new camera dangling heavily around her slender neck, eagerly snapping one shot after another. Her tiny frame is contradictory to the powerful spirit it embodies and those lucky enough to be welcomed into her guarded world are rarely left unchanged. Autumn sees the world and everything in it with an artistic and non-critical eye and anything she focuses her camera lens on becomes an untold story, from rusty old wheels and weathered buildings, to The Artist's most unusual creations.

We spent the entire afternoon traipsing over the massive sea rocks exposed by the low tide, her lens capturing colorful starfish clinging effortlessly to the sides, misplaced ladybugs wandering aimlessly over the damp sand, and a variety of shells and shiny smooth stones that dotted the winding shore. Watching her meld peacefully into the thick gray mist with the waves crashing over her tiny feet refreshed my gratitude for the honor of being her mother.

Late in the summer of 2009, The Taker had spared Autumn from a prescription addict with a death wish on Highway 200 in Montana, blessing us with a lingering season in her tangible presence and intensifying the love only a mother truly comprehends. The perfect afternoon melded into a perfect evening with her gentle spirit bouncing softly around our bubble's interior.

A scenic drive to Newport the next morning allowed Autumn to participate in choosing the perfect hot tub for her daddy, and although the skies were gray in Lincoln City, the sun shone brightly through the huge windows of the showroom that day in Newport, adding a supernatural sparkle to the tub we all had finally agreed upon. Autumn ran her slender fingers along the edge of the glittery finish, nodding in approval, her angelic frame bathed in a golden sunbeam and embedding another surreal snapshot into my memory. The owner of the shop was quick to offer resources for an electrician and a contractor that he was willing to contact on our behalf, and the door of the showroom closed behind us that afternoon with a promise of finalizing our purchase in the very near future.

The warm sunshine faded once again into a misty gray the closer we got to Lincoln City, creating a perfect opportunity for an afternoon trip through the bustling outlet mall to share in Autumn's passion for shopping. Billy and I sipped warm cocoa from a paper cup and enjoyed the simple pleasure of following close behind as she pointed out an eclectic array of unusual and colorful items that caught her attention along the way. Indulging her passion even further, we browsed shoulder-to-shoulder through several local tourist shops, and finished up the day with another buttery cup of Mo's chowder, snuggled up in a window seat watching the tide and fog roll into Siletz Bay.

Soon after Autumn flew away, Levi was scheduled to participate in a wilderness survival course on Mount Hood, along with two classmates. He was excited to spend four days on Oregon's most majestic and rugged mountain and we readily accepted the role of chauffeur, promising to deliver him promptly to the mountain and also back to the airport once his adventure came to an end. The class started early on a Thursday, and because we would be up before dawn, it took much convincing before Levi understood that we really were looking forward to the early morning drive. The beauty of the mountain at sunrise, along with Levi's easy smile and quick wit would be a perfect way to begin the day. We were not disappointed and laughed all the way up the mountain to Timberline Lodge where the infinite skyline was lit up with vibrant hues of sunrise.

We stood for a moment on the edge of the parking lot to take in the view of the many distant mountaintops jutting through thick morning clouds that were tinged with gold and scarlet far off in the distance. We each took one last breath of cleansing mountain air and zipped our sweatshirts against the early chill as we turned toward the lodge.

The lodge was built of large logs and local stone during the Great Depression and was also used as the exterior of the Overlook Hotel in the movie "The Shining." The lodge had fallen into disrepair early in the '50s but was brought back to life by a man named Richard Kohnstamm. He struggled for years, but soon turned a profit when skiing became popular in the 1950s and it is now owned by his son and continues to be a popular tourist destination throughout every season.

We bumped hip-to-hip through the lodge, taking in the many

historical displays while we searched for Levi's classroom. A selfish sigh escaped when a welcoming wave from a classmate caught Levi's eye, abruptly ending our tour. And with a quick kiss on my cheek followed by a wink, he turned to join his classmate and disappeared into the crowd. My breath always piles up in my throat for a split second whenever he turns to dive head first into life and leaves me waiting patiently on the shore. I already missed him and barely ten seconds had passed.

On our own once again, Billy and I stepped back out into the brisk morning air with intentions of exploring the grounds. The sun had barely peeked over the mountaintops and the air was still crisp and damp when we leashed Jazzy up for a quick hike. She immediately tugged at the end of her leash, sniffing everything in sight, with her curly tail wagging frantically as we meandered down several trails alongside the snowless ski slopes. Before long Billy began gathering a few perfect sticks from Mt. Hood to add to his collection, and he clumsily wrangled several into his arms before we made our way back up the steep side hill to the car. Jazzy's pace had slowed by the time she hopped onto her cozy backseat pillow, slurped down a long drink of water, turned a few circles and nested up a satisfactory napping spot.

A slow, winding drive back down the mountain with the windows down and the heavy scent of pine filling the entire car led us into the local diner in Government Camp, where we treated ourselves to a mid-morning breakfast of bacon and eggs. Energized by our freshly devoured meal and several cups of coffee that only a good diner can perfect, we started back up the mountain in search of the sign marked "Mirror Lake Trailhead" that had caught my attention on the opposite side of the highway. With wild abandon still driving me to squeeze in every adventure possible during that very significant summer, along with the hope of working off our calorie-laden breakfast, I parked the car. Guiding Billy and Jazzy over a wooden footbridge that crossed a roaring creek, we passed through the trailhead's entrance and into the shadowy forest of mammoth trees. For over an hour we zig-zagged up the narrow, musty mountain trail guarded by steep rock walls, past immense dislodged boulders and ancient moss covered trees. Once we'd painstakingly weaved our way to the top, we immediately began a trek back down the opposite side of the mountain through a narrow path of knee-high grass, and followed several wooden sign posts marking the way to the lake. Popping out of the forest we found the smooth, glistening surface of the water reflecting the mountain back to us like an intricate painting. The reason it was named Mirror Lake became readily apparent.

The tall grass nearly shielded several tents perched near the lake from view, and the tips of fishing poles bobbed just above the tall waving grass near the bank. From across the lake a few scantily clad teenagers could be seen stretched out on rickety little docks soaking up the fragrant mountain air and abundant sunshine. We stopped for a little while to let Jazzy rest and chatted with two young boys skipping stones on the water's still surface before we once again ducked into the cool shade of the forest and began the long winding hike back down to the car.

By the time we reached the parking lot it was mid-afternoon and the cool morning air had warmed with July's heat, so after Jazzy gulped down another pint or two of water, we put the windows down and took our time cruising over the winding road, darting in and out of the shadows, drenched in the intense scent of the forest and the soft warmth of summer air.

The weekend spent with Molly and the girls while we waited for Levi was entertaining and they were in the process of making a special dinner for him on Sunday evening when Billy and I were summoned back to the mountain. A short forty-five minutes later, we found ourselves back in Government Camp. While Levi's bags slid down one arm and into a heap in the trunk, he held out his opposite hand for the car keys, grinning a big dusty grin when I agreed to give up the driver's seat. Levi's six-foot frame towered over me, his bright blue eyes shining through the patches of dust embedded on his forehead and cheeks. His bright smile seemed to glow as he giggled, twisting his long legs into position beneath the steering wheel.

The last seat belt was barely snapped into place when he began to bubble over with enthusiasm, instantly drawing us into the multitude of emergency situations simulated during the course. Although his face was marked with fatigue, the skills and encouragement derived from his adventure were made evident as he passionately shared every detail. I quietly absorbed each word while my heart slowly puffed with pride from all he'd accomplished in a few short years and his eagerness to share it with us. Levi has a burning desire to deeply understand the complicated field of emergency medicine while also experiencing a variety of volunteer opportunities along the way; and, though not a natural part of his spiritual wardrobe, he consistently arms himself with the cloak of confidence necessary to succeed in his newly discovered world. His tenacity and bravery is a perfect match to Billy's, and with each heart-stopping step he took toward his plunge into deeper depths of the real world, I became more confident of his success and survival.

Levi was eager to shower away his mountain man appearance and indulge in Molly's home-cooked meal, while the chaos of Jamie's family filled the house with happy energy and the necessary medicine of laughter that we greedily devoured for hours.

Early the next morning, another kiss attached to a wink followed a promise to return again in August, before Levi disappeared through those same revolving airport doors.

CHAPTER 10

AUGUST ADVENTURES

WE USHERED JULY out and August in with preparations of a visit from my father, Papa, and his wife Donna. My mother had passed away more than a decade before, which devastated my father. Because Donna was somehow able to fill that unfillable void, it has left me with a deep respect for their relationship, and I looked forward to their visit with great anticipation. Papa had just recovered from a second close call with a heart attack and surgery to implant a pacemaker, but with his cardiologist's approval, he and Donna bravely embarked on the long journey by car, and my heart jumped when they finally called for directions to our bubble.

Because Papa's face wore the weariness of the long drive, I immediately settled them comfortably on the sofa, feet reclined and a cool drink in their hands. We set about making plans for their stay. Papa assured me he was up for a bit of sightseeing after a short rest and we started with a quick trip through the local tourist shops, followed by an afternoon drive to the historic Yaquina Head lighthouse just twenty miles south of Lincoln City.

We zipped our jackets up snugly under our chins and leaned into the strong westerly wind that greeted us when we stepped out of the car. Blinking away the tears welling up from the wind, I squinted to get a clear view of the long line of tourists winding far outside of the entrance in anticipation of climbing the one hundred and fourteen steps winding up to the top of Oregon's tallest lighthouse. Papa refused the long wait and the exhausting climb to the top, and we took in the view from behind the fence instead, near the steep and rugged edge of the huge basalt headland. A multitude of nesting sea birds flitting to and fro captured our attention while we scanned the surf far below in hopes of spotting a gray whale feeding in the shallow waters of summer. The whales had eluded us, and when we finally turned to follow the narrow path leading back to the parking lot, we found ourselves encircled by a medley of bright yellow and magenta wildflowers waving a graceful and colorful goodbye. While Papa slipped wearily into the back seat, Donna and I winked in agreement that his sightseeing adventures had come to an end for the day.

Papa is a slender, handsome man, and with little gray in his wavy dark hair he appeared much younger than his years. His kind blue eyes were the color of a summer sky and twinkled when he told an old joke that we had heard many times before. My heart ached for the sweet days of childhood when he seemed invincible. Yet it was comforting to spend the evening sharing a bottle of wine and ancient jokes, now known throughout the family as Papa-*isms*. But the twinkle in his eyes quickly dimmed with fatigue, signaling his desire to say goodnight.

Donna, too, was eager to experience the Pacific Ocean at low tide in hopes of filling her camera with colorful photos of abundant starfish. But, the next morning I feared that Papa would not have the strength required to trudge through the heavy sand while battling a harsh and chilly wind. Papa was determined though, and prepared to make the long trek all the way from the beach access to Cascade Head and back again. Billy loved his beach walks and proudly handed Papa and Donna each a walking stick before we began a slow and steady pace to the tide pools.

Donna's excitement while she tip-toed over the rocks in search of starfish and other unexpected tide pool inhabitants was infectious, but the journey had taken a toll on Papa and his usual rosy cheeks were far too pale by the time we finally reached the car. I quickly had him reclining on the sofa again for a few hours of recovery time.

Our wedding anniversary and Donna's birthday both fell on that same weekend, so while Papa rested, I prepared a feast of grilled salmon, bowls of ripe green peas, blueberries picked fresh from our little garden, and his favorite dessert of coconut cream pie. Papa and my Billy laughed together, drank wine, and devoured the creamy sweet pie. Donna and I watched and smiled. Another snapshot was recorded.

I had become far too aware of fleeting bits of time, and soon Papa and Donna were stowing their luggage and promising to check in often as they made their way to Idaho where they would visit Papa's sisters before making the long trip back to Montana. I prayed another silent prayer that our visit had not been a *last time*.

Less than a week later, my youngest brother, Clint, and his adventurous wife, Lisa, made the long drive to deliver a car we had been forced to leave behind during the big move. Once again, the abundant sunshine we had enjoyed in June was elusive in August and their visit was riddled with powerful winds and heavy gray skies. They, too, anticipated a beachcombing trip, so shortly after their arrival, walking sticks and camera in hand, we mastered another trip to Cascade Head through steady, strong winds. Treasures were found and photos were taken.

Clint's passion for fishing surpasses Billy's by far and a deep-sea fishing trip had been scheduled even before they left Montana, so before dawn the next morning we set out for Depoe Bay to embark on an adventure aboard a giant chartered vessel. We had all wisely taken medication with breakfast to ward off sea-sickness and crossed our fingers that it would be effective while we took inventory of our soda crackers and water bottles in the cabin once we boarded. The howling winds forced crashing waves to pound the side of the boat when we passed through the narrow gate of the bay and into open waters, forcing us to hold tightly to whatever stable part of the ship we could find while the captain bucked monstrous waves out to even deeper waters. After what seemed like hours of painfully enduring wave after wave, the captain finally announced that we were pausing to drop crab pots. We had purchased the option of snaring crab too, and each participant would be allowed twelve Dungeness crab should the pots retrieved later that day contain our legal limit. A quick mental tally of twelve times the four of us left me wondering what we would do with forty-eight crab. I was still pondering this when we arrived at the captain's lucky fishing spot and he began to bark clear-cut instructions over the loudspeaker on how to drop the baited hook and the exact time to reel it back up. Once our lines were dropped as instructed, we held tightly to our rods while bracing ourselves against the side of the boat, rocking nauseatingly to and fro as the wind and mist bit at our cheeks and we waited patiently for a strike from the ocean depths. Several others on the boat were already calling for the captain's deckhand, and one had even caught a ling cod before any of us even felt our first strike.

While waiting to hook a big one, I noticed a few of the other passengers had gotten seasick and were lurching over the side of the boat with dreadful expressions pasted painfully over their pale faces. About the same time, Lisa also hung far over the edge of the boat and then quickly ran down to the cabin below the fishing deck. I left Billy, now appearing a bit hypothermic, under Clint's watchful eye while I went down to check on Lisa. I found her in the cabin nibbling on soda crackers that held the sickness at bay. Before long we were once again manning our posts back on deck, ready to reel in a big one. Billy had been shivering uncontrollably, and just as we were about to set our poles down again so I could lead him into the warmth of the cabin, he felt the familiar tug of a strike on his line. Soon after he pulled up his strange looking sea bass, we each had the thrill of reeling in our first catch too. Although we had hoped to hook a big ling cod, several sea bass were all we reeled in before the captain instructed us to stow away our poles for the rough journey back to the crab pots.

We again gripped whatever secure part of the ship we could find and held on tightly while the captain bucked the waves back to where the crab pots were dropped a few hours earlier. Still wondering what to do with that much crab, I watched as the pots were pulled up one by one and the keepers were tallied. Indeed, it was a good day for crabbing, and Billy giggled when the deck hand announced that forty-eight freshly caught crab belonged to us. We were relieved to learn that for just one dollar per crab, they would clean and cook our bounty back at the dock. That left us with the final task of cracking the crab and teasing the delicate and sweet morsels of meat from their backs and legs, which took three long hours once we got back home. With the kitchen finally cleaned up and the aromatic bags of empty shells stowed safely outside, we admired our abundance of fresh crab meat and sea bass filets. Wearing proud grins we congratulated each other on surviving a full day of wild abandon.

Our pancakes and coffee the next morning were exceptionally satisfying, while we laughed and relived our adventure. We spent the relaxing afternoon blending with tourists while browsing through the local shops lining Highway 101, and finished up with dinner and grown-up beverages at a cozy local tavern. My scrapbook of snap-shots continued to grow.

Time melted away, and Billy and I soon watched as Clint turned the rental car onto the highway and they disappeared into the sun-shine that had eluded us during their stay. It was comforting to know that Billy had a final appointment scheduled with the nurse practitio-ner in Montana, and in a few short weeks we would see them again.

I had been anxiously awaiting Billy's upcoming September ap-pointment in Montana, hoping for a recommendation and referral to a neurologist nearer our new home as she had previously prom-ised. Something had to be done to quiet the monster's persistent roar. Maybe there were new drugs that would slow down those damn proteins growing like weeds in his beautiful brain. He barely spoke, and caring for himself had gotten worse far too quickly. I had been gripped with fear for the past few weeks while the renewed sparkle in his blue eyes continued to dim. With childlike dependency he began looking to me for affirmation and assistance with nearly every task, eventually retreating more frequently to the solitude of the garage to strip his sticks while his favorite music tempered the frustration so apparent on his handsome face.

The helplessness welling up inside of me intensified when I read the words in an unexpected and impersonal letter from the nurse practitioner while walking back from the mailbox one damp afternoon. A straightforward explanation of early retirement in order to spend quality time with her already retired husband, finished up with the recommendation that we visit a family doctor of our choosing, as Billy's condition was stable and the need for a neurologist was no longer necessary. Her flippant use of the word *stable* echoed in my mind as I recalled his *un*stable and *un*predictable behavior over the past weeks, and it left me feeling completely alone in the midst of our escalating war. Her hidden meaning, disguised by professional jargon, allowed hopelessness to gain a forceful grip around my chest, and with Billy's pendulous changes fresh in my mind, I once again struggled to catch my breath.

Billy seemed completely unaffected by the news and agreed to see whichever family doctor I suggested. I flipped through the yellow pages and jotted down the number to a local clinic that advertised more than one internal medicine doctor. One quick phone call left us with a new patient appointment two weeks later. I began to pray for an intelligent and compassionate professional to lead us through each frightening battle now hovering on the nearby horizon.

The apprehension of starting over with a new doctor was temporarily relieved by Levi's final visit before the fall semester began. He and his Uncle Jamie had participated in the Hood to Coast relay every August during his undergraduate years, and without much training he had reluctantly agreed to join the team again. His arrival two weeks before the relay allowed time for several runs on the beach in hopes of increasing his stamina, and also allowed him to accompany Billy and me to our appointment with the new doctor that I had spontaneously and randomly chosen. From the moment Levi arrived I began to draw from his endless supply of optimism that immediately illuminated our gloomy bubble.

We located the clinic with time to spare and after completing a stack of required new-patient paperwork, we flipped through old magazines and giggled at Levi's comical remarks about celebrity related headlines adorning most of the magazine covers. A few minutes later, we were whispering from our corner of the exam room while the nurse recorded Billy's vital signs and requested pertinent information for his newly created file. When Dr. O., a very tall and soft-spoken man, quietly entered and introduced himself, an involuntary sigh of relief escaped. I watched him shake Billy's hand first, and then Levi's. His kind eyes expressed the compassion I had been praying for and the helplessness I had been harboring slowly began to lift a bit. He reviewed Billy's records, answered questions, and assured us that he had professional connections with a prominent neurologist in the nearby city of Corvallis. However, he patiently explained that Billy was still being treated with the *only* drugs available, and that expensive trips to a neurologist would be an unnecessary source of anxiety for both of us. But it was his pessimism regarding my renewed interest in clinical trials that allowed helplessness to engulf me once again, while his unspoken words mimicked those of the now retired nurse practitioner in Montana. They had both silently made it clear that Billy's monster was gaining ground and the medications would not prevent its advance. The fear accompanying that harsh reality swallowed up any glimmer of hope I had been clinging to. Relief that we had found a kind and helpful doctor, combined with Levi's protective arm draped over my shoulder when we left the clinic, made it possible to temporarily squelch the fear spreading like a wildfire inside of me.

Much of the afternoon had been left unplanned and in an attempt to brighten the mood, I suggested a quick trip to the hot tub shop in Newport to finalize the purchase of the shimmering hot tub we had chosen during Autumn's visit. It did not take much convincing, and before long we were visiting with Robyn, the robust and friendly owner of the spa shop again. Robyn had a down-to-earth quality about him that left us feeling as if we had known him for many years, and because he looked Billy directly in the eye when he spoke and included him in the thrill of the purchase, it endeared me to him even further. He also shook Levi's hand and allowed him to ask the questions Billy was unable to articulate. Billy followed along, nodding as though he were fully understanding the conversation, yet fumbling over the simplest words when he became brave enough to join in. Watching him struggle, I found myself intrigued once again. He seemed to understand our words as they passed through the tangles, but they would disappear into the maze, leaving his thoughts scrambled in the shadows. His face grimaced. He giggled an embarrassed giggle, muttered, "Never mind," and turned to look out the showroom window.

We left a down payment for the tub and agreed to have Robyn contact an electrician and a contractor to pour the concrete. The trip to Newport had done its job and the raging fire of fear that began the day had been reduced to smoldering coals for the time being. Confident that Billy's hot tub would be the focal point of our back yard very soon, we immediately turned our attention to the real purpose of Levi's visit. The Hood to Coast relay would be an exciting distraction.

Just before dawn a few days later, Jamie was shaking Levi awake and taunting him about his youthful, yet out-of-shape body, while reminding him that he was scheduled for the first leg of the relay. He returned jabs at his middle-aged uncle as he ran fingers through his wild morning hair and stumbled toward the coffee pot while checking new messages on his cell phone. I dropped them off at the team's designated meeting spot. Then we all began the long wait between updates while he and Jamie alternated legs of the relay with teammates over the next thirty-six hours.

The Hood to Coast Relay was started in 1982 by Bob Foote, a Portland area architect and president of the Oregon Road Runners Club. The family-owned business began aggressive fundraising for cancer research after its founder was diagnosed and treated for melanoma, and it remains one of the largest road race, cancer fundraising programs in the nation.

The course of the relay is nearly two hundred miles long and begins from the parking lot of Timberline Lodge on the slopes of Mount Hood, continues through the city of Portland, over the Oregon Coast Range, and into the historic beach town of Seaside.

Each twelve person team is allowed two van-sized vehicles to follow in support of their runners. Those vehicles are often flamboyantly decorated with the team's name and silly themes to match, and winners for the best team name, best decorations, best team outfits and outstanding volunteers are announced at the awards ceremony on the sandy beaches of Seaside after the race ends on Saturday night.

Billy and I were thrilled to return to the same quaint beach town where we had honeymooned and began our brand new life together just a heartbeat ago. I rested my head back into the endless summer sky, melding into the whoosh of the ocean while the hot August sun warmed the sand we were comfortably burying our feet in. The memories flooding my mind slowly faded as a growing crowd of runners and spectators began to spill over the promenade and onto the bustling beach.

It wasn't long before Jamie and Levi limped past the finish line with their team and disappeared into the sea of party-goers that were prepared to celebrate the event long into the night. We met up with our weary runners in the beer garden and watched with amusement as they quenched their thirst, filled their bellies with lunch from the food vendor's tent, and relived every hilarious event that had occurred over the past two days they had shared together. An amused smile lit up Billy's face as he watched the interaction between his brother and his son, and although his occasional attempts to join the conversation were slow and difficult, the smile remained right up until he sighed and closed his eyes for the two-hour drive back to Lincoln City later that evening.

Jamie and Molly landed in our bubble with us after the relay with a plan to launch Billy's boat into the Siletz River the next day and catch a few fresh Dungeness crab on our own. Levi would take an early flight back to Arizona the next morning, and though he was disappointed that he would not be able to experience the adventure of crabbing, he eagerly helped Jamie and Billy prepare the boat for our maiden voyage into Oregon waters. They stowed the crab rings, charged the boat's batteries, and packed up the bait as Molly and I gathered rain jackets, warm clothes, and prepared plenty of snacks. The morning was charged with excitement and after devouring an energy-packed breakfast, Levi waved a disappointed goodbye and began his journey back to school.

The owner of the local marina on the Siletz River was in the business of renting crab rings, but was less than enthusiastic when we coerced him into a beginner's tutorial on crabbing. We antagonized him with questions on how to properly secure raw chicken drumsticks into mesh bait bags and how to safely navigate the Siletz River and avoid the dangers of the bay. His gruff tutorial ended with a stern warning to be back before the tide retreated later that day or risk having the boat stranded on a stretch of exposed silt and sand.

The rest of the day was guided by the clock as we maneuvered down the river as instructed, hunting for fertile crabbing grounds. We dropped pots, waited patiently in hopes of ravenous Dungeness crab sauntering into our snares, and pulled them up time and again. All the while I watched as Jamie repeatedly showed Billy how to pull straight up on the rope, not allowing the pot to drag, and then drew him into the thrill of separating the keepers from the throwbacks. Laughter filled the air when several throwbacks escaped into the boat and chaos ensued in an attempt to tackle and toss the speedy crustaceans back into the bay without getting a finger caught between the pinchers of their powerful claws.

A bank of thick clouds had blocked the sun's warmth and a steady and chilly breeze had blown throughout the afternoon, so it was no surprise that Ashley shrieked with delight from beneath her fort of cozy blankets when Jamie announced that the tide had begun to suck water back into the Pacific and it was time to stow the pots. Our full day's bounty was small compared to our deep sea trip, but we were filled with pride at our success when we pulled our last string of pots out of the frigid water and tallied our catch. Recalling the threat of being stranded in the deep silt of the Siletz River at low tide, we puttered up close to the dock where its rapid retreat had already left a narrow slip of water barely deep enough to load the boat back onto the trailer.

Once we got back home, Jamie and Billy hosed off the salt and seaweed clinging to every inch of the boat, and Molly and I filled giant pots of heavily salted water. While the water began to bubble, we all watched an internet tutorial on cooking and cleaning Dungeness crab several times. Then, with their front claws pinching wildly, we forced the struggling crabs one by one into the rapidly boiling water, watching as their murky brown shells turned instantly to a bright scarlet. The tutorial was watched once more before we cleaned the crab and prepared to sit down and tease tender morsels once again from the hard shells of the claws and backs. It had been a distracting and exciting weekend, and our next attempt at wild abandon would be in the deep and fertile waters of Garibaldi Bay.

CHAPTER 11

FINISHING TOUCHES

WITH SUMMER'S END inching closer, we were thrilled when, just as Robyn had promised, an electrician called shortly after our visit to Newport and, in just one afternoon, installed the electrical lines required to power our tub. A few days later, we received a phone call from Ryan, a self-employed contractor who stopped by near the end of a long work day to estimate the labor and materials necessary to pour the concrete patio. He took his time measuring and jotting down ideas before he gave us his final suggestion along with estimated costs of materials and labor. Ryan embodied many of the same qualities I respect in my three brothers, which put me at ease right away. We readily accepted his offer to begin the project as soon as his schedule allowed.

With a plan in place and his workday finished, a relaxed grin finally replaced the gruff business expression Ryan had held for the past hour. He reached out a dusty hand for the beer I offered, stayed awhile and patiently answered questions Billy struggled to ask about salmon fishing in the local rivers.

It wasn't long before Ryan arrived with a crew of rough-looking concrete specialists who set about shoveling the uneven mounds of clay soil in the backyard into a level surface for the patio. The heat and humidity prevailed throughout the day and wheelbarrows filled with giant clods of clay were wheeled through the gate and spilled into the forest. With a final warning from the foreman to stay inside, the back yard was soon laden with yards of freshly poured concrete being smoothed and tamped into a flawless finish.

I immediately locked the patio door leading to the backyard, looked directly into Billy's eyes, both hands firmly planted on his shoulders, and said,

"Billy, I have locked the doors because the concrete outside is wet. Please don't let Jazzy outside. Okay? Do you understand? Please don't open that door."

I pointed at the door. He nodded, and stuttered,

"Yes, yes. Yes! I get it! I won't open the door!"

In keeping with the predictability of *un*predictable behavior that was part of the Alzheimer's package, Billy promptly forgot his promise to stay indoors. Within ten minutes he felt the need to check on the progress of the crew, and opened the patio door leading directly to the freshly troweled surface of wet concrete. Jazzy took full advantage of the opportunity to protect her home against the big, bad concrete crew and barreled past Billy. With a final threatening leap off of the porch steps, she landed with all four paws into the shiny smooth surface of the concrete and directly into the face of the sweaty, worn-out foreman.

All of the crew was aware of Billy's mischievous monster, and the foreman's gnarled frown quickly dissolved when he saw Billy, his hands pressed into his head, and a horrified expression contorting his entire face. I reached Jazzy just as she flipped around, shook wet concrete everywhere, flew back through the open patio door, and continued to fling more wet clumps all over the dining room walls and furniture. The situation quickly turned hilarious and once the laughter had subsided, and both Billy and Jazzy had recovered from the horror of it, the foreman grinned and smoothed the concrete to perfection once again.

The need to find a way of melding the love I felt for Billy as my husband and best friend, to the new love I felt for him as my childlike dependent was confounding. My emotions became muddled through a continual comparison of his current childlike state to that of our children when they were small. I had become vigilantly aware of dangers, realizing that his degree of understanding and remembering were continually changing, and unlike that of a child who would learn by experience, Billy would quickly forget, rendering warnings or reminders futile.

The weary crew worked late into the afternoon, and finally transformed the disheveled back yard into the anticipated, but not-yet-firm-enough-to-bear-our-weight patio that we had envisioned. We were now even more impatient to indulge in the swirling warm water of our new tub under a misty night sky filled with stars, so we called Robyn to confirm the tub's delivery date. Waiting on delivery of our tub, and the ten days required for the concrete to cure, left a perfect window of time for a trip back to Montana before we *hunkered down* for the winter, as Billy referred to it.

CHAPTER 12

THE GREAT MOOSE'S TOUR

DUE TO THE unexpected resignation of the nurse practitioner back in Montana, the trip we had planned for September no longer had the pressure of a scheduled arrival date, and we began preparations for a scenic road trip back home, intending to visit family and friends all along the way. When we agreed to spend some time in Kalispell with Grandma Judi and her sweetheart, Jack, Billy shot me a sly grin and dubbed the trip "The Great Moose's Tour."

Judi held a secure and revered place in Billy's heart and adoration consumed his face at the mere mention of her name over the years. Judi and Billy's father were married shortly after he and Joyce divorced, and although Judi was already full-time mother to Billy's sisters, she had also graciously accepted Billy and his younger brother, Rick, into her home when they chose to leave Oregon during their adolescent years.

Being left on her own, Joyce had often struggled to balance work and life as a single mother of four boys; and because Billy and Rick were older, they were often allowed freedoms young boys can rarely manage with discernment. Billy was barely into his teenage years when he traded his dangerous freedom for the structured and disciplined environment Judi sternly provided once they lived under their father's roof in Montana. Billy believed that Judi had saved him. Although humility does not allow her to claim the title as Billy's savior, he believed she was.

Kalispell is home to the world famous Moose's Saloon, and Billy had spent many a long summer night there filled with the wild abandon of youth. The saloon's dimly lit interior is crowded with bulky wooden tables, bar tops, and beams that have been marred over the years by travelers, local patrons, and sweethearts who have carved their names deep into the thick rugged surfaces of the wood. A layer of sawdust and discarded peanut shells cover the floor, and the faceless laughter of beer drinkers and pizza eaters echoes from within the dark shadows. There, deep in the heart of Montana, my Billy had stored an album of memories in the recesses of his mind, filled with adventures and extravagant irresponsibility.

Many of those adventures included Woody, who grew up in Kalispell and had become one of Billy's closest friends through his job at Buttrey Foods in Great Falls. And although for months to years at a time when Billy and Woody went their separate ways, the brotherly affection they held for one another often brought them back together with a comfortable ease. Woody and his wife, Beth, became an important part of our lives as our young families grew, and life's sorrows and responsibilities solidified our friendship. The special relationship between Woody and Beth was also one to be admired as we observed the courage that strengthened their love into one that would be forever unshakable, when in the early years of their marriage Woody was diagnosed with viral myocarditis, and a few short years later The Taker claimed their second child at just three months old. Their respect for one another was an example to me whenever the struggles of marriage caused visions of freedom to infiltrate my selfish bones in those early years of marital adjustment. So, with twenty-six years comfortably behind us, running with Billy through that particular field of youthful memories filled me with joyful anticipation, and Moose's Saloon quickly became the cornerstone of our travels.

Moose and Shirley Miller opened Moose's Saloon in 1957, the same year that Billy was born, and in the early seventies they expanded their business to include a shop of memoirs. During one of those early visits to the saloon, Billy had purchased a cap with their logo and year of his birth which he had treasured for many years. That old cap had been looking pretty tattered and he made it emphatically clear that he intended to replace his old Moose's Saloon cap with a crisp new one, as well as quenching his thirst bellied up to the same bar where he had shared many cold beers and good times with young friends so long ago. The mischievous grin he couldn't hide when he attempted to share a bit of their glory days at Moose's Saloon almost made up for the lack of sparkle in his ocean blue eyes while he stumbled over words and I did what I could to fill in the blanks. The puzzle pieces of each story fell slowly into place, and when Billy's laughter filled the room the joy of the moment could not be contained. I had always envied the way he managed to live every moment of his young life with such passion and lack of regret. The memories driving "The Great Moose's Tour," and my unspoken realization that it could simultaneously be the first *and the last* annual event, gave our adventure a much deeper meaning. And so, I greedily absorbed every second of Billy's enthusiasm as he reached deep into the vault of long term memories and did his best to share them with me.

A slow tour through stunning Glacier Park would include a toe-tingling climb up and over its infamous *Going-to-the-Sun Road*, and I filed away a mental map of our trip and immediately got busy packing and loading the trunk with road-trip essentials that evening. I snuggled up even tighter than usual to Billy when we slipped into bed, and with the warmth of his breath caressing my shoulder, I drifted into peaceful sleep, eager to soak up every decadent moment of "The Great Moose's Tour."

Daybreak soon poured a shower of gold through the window blinds, and in no time I had buckled Billy safely in as co-pilot with Jazzy perched proudly on the console between the front seats, panting and wagging her curly tail wildly when we turned into the shaded tunnel beneath the towering trees on Pacific Highway 101. With the rising sun winking through the branches and our steaming coffee melting away the morning chill, "The Great Moose's Tour" was underway.

A quick stop for a goodbye hug before we set out found Molly's kitchen smelling of warm toast and coffee. She greeted us with a full creamy cup in the midst of the morning bustle of a school day. Jamie and Molly have a constant infectious air of energy that unintentionally poured over Billy and me and we were suddenly even more ready to hit the open road with a goal of filling our souls with joy and sunshine.

With a wave goodbye, we donned our sunglasses and headed east toward The Dalles. Just half an hour later, we pulled into the crowded and familiar parking lot that sits at the foot of Multnomah Falls. We had rarely passed up the opportunity to behold the magnificence of the falls, and the morning sunshine allowed it to be a perfect beginning to our trip.

A steady, thunderous roar from the 620-foot cascade of icy water, pouring over a towering wall of rock, echoed through the captivated crowd of on-lookers when we joined them at its base. And just past the historic Multnomah Lodge, we climbed the wide, crowded stairway toward a steep trail leading through the damp forest to Benson's Bridge, which spans the first tier of the falls. Benson's Bridge was built in 1914 by Simon Benson, a prominent Portland businessman and one of the builders of the old Columbia highway. We wound our way up the trail, and from the center of the bridge, we stood before the dynamic power spilling over the mountaintop above us, and took in the nerve-tingling view of the pool far below. The heavy spray of the falls poured a chilly mist over us while we stood once again in silent awe of its majestic beauty.

Native American lore tells the story of a sickness that fell upon the Multnomah people and, believing that the Great Spirit was angry with them, a very old medicine man told his people that the sacrifice of a young maiden would save them. When the daughter of the chief found her lover sick with fever, she followed the trail to the river and climbed to the top of the rocks. She asked the Great Spirit for a sign in the sky, and when she saw the moon rising over the river, she raised her arms to the Great Spirit and threw herself over the edge of the cliff. When the sickness lifted the next morning they went in search of the missing maiden and found her dead. The chief prayed to the Great Spirit asking for assurance that his daughter's life was not sacrificed in vain. The people looked up to see a stream of silvery white pour over the cliff and form a floating mist at their feet, and the stream of white grew into the high and powerful waterfall. The legend says that the spirit of the beautiful maiden visits the place of her brave sacrifice during the winter months, and she stands all dressed in white amongst the trees near the falls.

The lore and beauty of Multnomah Falls leaves me quiet after each visit, and in silence, hand-in-hand, Billy and I made our way back to the parking lot. It was a perfect beginning to our journey.

Not far into the Columbia Gorge a sign that Billy had pointed out to me many times over the years caught my attention. It said "Vista House – Open," which is not always the case. I immediately added it to our tour. A quick turn-around on the interstate and an exit shortly thereafter found us winding our way up a steep and narrow, well-worn road that seemed to go on forever. Just as we were thinking we may be lost, the dark tunnel of the forest burst into a vast and sun-filled parking lot bordering a rock wall that separated visitors from the dangerous cliffs below. We pulled into one of the many vacant spots and leashed Jazzy up for a quick walk before we began our next sightseeing adventure. In recent weeks, Billy had often appeared unusually awestruck at the Earth's natural beauty, and I watched his expression light up while he quietly whispered "Wow!" and took in the mighty Columbia River and the golden morning shining on the valley far below. I watched and pondered, wondering if stirrings deep inside of his beautiful brain had somehow altered his senses, perhaps magnifying the vibrant colors of the Earth and the majesty of the mountains, rivers, and sky. Or had the habitual hurried pace of his previous life simply prevented appreciation of the artistry that had always been right before him?

With Jazzy nestled safely back in the car, we made our way to the Vista House, so named by Samuel Lancaster, who in 1913 supervised the Columbia River Highway project hoping to make the wonder of the Columbia River Gorge accessible to travelers. He thought Crown Point was the ideal site for "an observatory from which the view both up and down the Columbia could be viewed in silent communion with the infinite."

The octagonal exterior of the building wears a covering of gray sandstone and boasts a green tile roof. Once inside, we found sheets of Alaskan marble covering the floors and stairs, and fascinating architecture and history met us at every turn. There was even a gift shop and espresso bar that lured us in as we browsed and took in breathtaking views past the numerous floor-to-ceiling windows. My spirit soared as I watched Billy meander slowly throughout this place of intrigue indulging in its historic beauty before we entered the confines of the car once again. The peace of the morning had replaced Billy's recent anxious mood with quiet contentment, and he relaxed into his seat while Bob Dylan's *Tangled Up in Blue* poured through the speakers and filled the empty space around us.

We wound our way through the Gorge, warmed by the sun's intensity filtering through the windshield, and I reached over and squeezed Billy's hand as I often did. But this time he gave me a cozy squeeze back and topped it off with the special wink he reserved just for me. A tiny bit of my old Billy surfaced and it lit up my world. That wink fueled me all the way to the junction near Missoula that marked our way to Seeley Lake.

Billy had several past colleagues he wanted to say hello to during our trip and one in particular was now managing a local hardware store in the little mountain town of Seeley Lake, Montana. Pat was unaware that we were in the store and a smile warmed his face the moment he saw Billy. They spent awhile catching up and Pat was careful in his conversation, giving Billy time to comprehend and respond slowly. I could tell by Pat's expression that he was saddened by Billy's sudden and obvious progression, yet pleased with the opportunity to hash over old times if only briefly. Billy was thrilled to revisit an era in his career long gone with someone who understood, and he held a partial smile the rest of the way to Kalispell. I secretly wished that all of his old friends could have kept in touch over the years. Billy would often sing, hilariously off key, the lyrics of the Neil Young song, *"One of these days, I'm gonna sit down and write a long letter, to all the good friends I've known."*

Although, he would also grin and quote, *"I've got plenty of friends and the fun never ends, as long as I'm buyin'."*

Billy's friends meant the world to him.

Grandma Judi and Jack had been expecting us and were generous with their hospitality. Jack treated us to a night out at an Italian restaurant where my Billy tried wild boar for the first time and was pleasantly surprised at the tender and flavorful morsel. Judi was also able to accompany us to Moose's Saloon the next afternoon where Billy's wish to indulge in a cold beer and buy a crisp new cap was realized. Mission accomplished. "The Great Moose's Tour" had been a success, and for two more glorious days, we puttered around Kalispell with Judi, and late into the evenings enjoyed stories of Jack's days in the Navy.

Billy handed out gifts of freshly-crafted walking sticks before we buckled up and set our sights on the majestic Rocky Mountains and a slow and peaceful drive through Glacier Park.

Our first stop was Apgar Village, tucked away at the southern end of Lake McDonald just two miles north of West Glacier, and host to several quaint souvenir shops where tourists can fill up on Rocky Mountain air and huckleberry ice cream. We leashed up Jazzy and stretched our legs, filling our lungs with the scent of home.

Lake McDonald was picturesque and the icy water crystal clear, allowing us to see the many multi-colored stones covering the shallow bottom near the water's edge. Billy picked up several musty sticks during our walk along the lakeshore, tapping each one on the soft dirt and discarding several before carefully choosing a fairly straight one to tuck into the trunk. Keeping a vigilant eye for quality sticks had become an obsession of Billy's, and once we left Apgar Village, I found myself slowing down to a snail's pace as we worked our way through the mountains just in case he spotted a good one and insisted we pull over to inspect it. The absolute joy he found in spying a perfect stick from the mountains of Montana, with a hope of turning it into a work of art, filled me with overwhelming love and I could never turn down his request to stop and wriggle the mud- and moss-covered gem into the trunk right next to our luggage.

It took much of the afternoon to slowly wind our way up the dangerously narrow Going-to-the-Sun Road, and over its peak at Logan's Pass where it crosses the Continental Divide. One of the few safe turnouts along the way allowed us to stop and take photos. A backdrop of immense mountain peaks was still tipped in bits of winter's white, dropping vertically through a thick forest of pine to the rambling river below. Billy stood near the steep edge and patiently allowed me to take one beautiful snapshot after another.

It didn't take very long to wind our way back down the opposite side of the steep road, and a sigh of relief mixed with disappointment escaped my lips when the mountains disappeared in the rear view mirror and the flat Montana prairie stretched out for miles before us. Recent years have left me with a newfound appreciation for the beauty of the Montana prairie, but it could never compare to the grandeur of the Rocky Mountains.

Cut Bank, Montana, our next planned stop, is known as the coldest spot in the nation, and more often than not swirling dirt devils are roaring through the town and back out over the vast prairie. In this dusty rural town another previous colleague Billy had grown fond of managed the local Albertson's store and he was adamant about stopping by to say hello to Mario. We did. Mario was very busy, but grinned a handsome grin and gave Billy a few moments of his time. Mario had taken Billy under his wing during a business trip the previous year, just as the monster had begun to rumble. It could have been dangerous, and I often wonder what must have been going through Mario's mind during that snowy March meeting in Minneapolis when Billy had trouble finding his way around the hotel on his own. The rumors must have been abundant on the corporate grapevine and my inability to protect him at that time was frightening.

We shared a sandwich in the car before we left, but the silence was suffocating. It had not been so long ago when Billy was also a respected part of the management team and his solemn expression made me wonder if his visit with Mario had magnified his current level of inability. I had clung to his strength and determination during his career, and prayed through the heavy silence for the bravery I would now need to be his lifeline when the monster's appetite became insatiable.

Jazzy finally broke the quiet when she tipped my open bottle of chocolate milk all over herself in the back seat, setting off chaos as we scrambled to mop up the mess with a few paper towels rolling around on the floor boards. With order restored, we turned onto the highway with hopes of reaching the next stop in Choteau before dark.

Choteau is nearly an hour and a half south of Cut Bank and often referred to as *The Gateway to the Rocky Mountain Front*. Billy's long-time friend, Danny, and his wife, Kathy, relocated there from Havre when corporate nonsense caused them to re-evaluate the importance of peace over monetary reward once their children were grown. The quiet beauty of their quaint Montana town, complete with the Rocky Mountains standing guard in the west, must have been a comforting perk to offset the angst of their life-changing decisions. Billy and Danny had spent many weekends together fishing for walleye on Tiber Reservoir or telling fish tales in either one of their garages whenever they had a rare day off together. We were looking forward to catching up on lost time throughout the softness of a warm summer evening.

We were greeted at the garden gate with smiles and a beautiful sunset gleaming brilliant rays of scarlet and fluorescent orange over the rugged peaks behind us as we wrestled our luggage out of the trunk and Danny guided us past Kathy's colorful beds of flowers and his meticulously manicured lawn. Kathy had been putting finishing touches on a feast of enchiladas and I indulged in her friendship while she tidied up the kitchen once they were in the oven. It didn't take Danny long to put a glass of wine in Billy's hand and set him down in a comfortable chair next to him at the patio table. I followed Kathy through the screen door and ran face first into a cloud of cigarette smoke that Danny had been puffing into the dusky air. The familiar scent of tobacco engulfed me and I breathed in the nostalgia as deeply as I could. Danny was fully aware of Billy's monster and chatted long, but was also kind and pretended to understand when Billy joined in through broken sentences and apologies for lost trains of thought. Billy would chuckle and make a silly face, but uncomfortable sympathy became an unwelcome guest that lingered for the remainder of the evening.

We devoured Kathy's warm, bubbly dinner of cheesy enchiladas, savored the sweetness of the wine, and finally said our goodnights. Wrapped up in the comfort of each other, a bit of moonlight peered through sheer drapes and bathed Billy's weary face in a ghostly shade of pale. I relaxed into his warmth and the music of his heart, while the fullness of the day slowly faded.

Morning rose quickly and it took more energy than usual to ready us both for the last leg of our journey. Extra time had become necessary for that which was no longer second nature to the stubbornly independent husband I had grown so fond of over the years, and frustration had begun to make a frequent appearance. My attempt to slip Billy's t-shirt over his head and wriggle his fists through the sleeves caused my heart to sink when my mind again flashed back to the days when I wrestled Levi and Autumn's little arms into their shirt sleeves too. The familiar fire of fear snuffed my breath, drained my face of life's blood and nearly buckled my knees beneath me while I watched my Billy twist and tug at the end of his belt, struggling to fasten it through the buckle. I clenched my fists and refrained from stepping in to ease his struggle, because he always seemed relieved and a bit proud when he finished anything all on his own. Tears once again sat threateningly on the edge of my lids, but I forced them back and let him see only a proud smile when he patted his freshly fastened belt with satisfaction and shot me a confident grin. His cheerfulness sucked the color back into my cheeks and I locked my elbow with his and turned him toward the door. We were off to breakfast and the now routine regimen of medication that I prayed would quiet the monster.

By the time we reached the kitchen and found Danny gazing out the window dressed and ready for work, I was wondering if I would have the energy to finish the day and it was barely eight o'clock in the morning. He pointed the way to the coffee pot and gave us a grumpy old man, "Good morning."

Danny has a pensive, pondering nature at times, but a snarky retort forced a chuckle out of him and perked me up at the same time. It was a work day for both Dan and Kathy, and after a quick cup of coffee we were ready to tuck the bags and Jazzy back into the car. Great Falls was a quick forty-five minutes away and we were both eager to be home, even for just a few days.

The cottonwood trees planted during my youth now shrouded the house from view and formed a shadowy tunnel glowing with fall's palette when we turned into the driveway. We were being drawn into a colorful painting, and I inched over the railroad tracks, slowing the car in a wishful attempt to slow time too. Golden leaves of autumn danced past the windshield and swirled around our feet when we finally opened the door and set them down on familiar ground.

Although we knew it was a workday and no one would be inside, an unexpected and eerie silence hung heavily in the stagnant air, boldly greeting us when we creaked open the door to find my lifeless childhood home overwhelmingly empty. Melancholy and I wandered from room to room of the large, now thunderously quiet, house that once bustled daily with the lively chatter and chaos of thirteen grandchildren when Papa and Grandma Rose lived there. I allowed my mind to momentarily revisit all of the holidays, noisy dinners, and rambunctious birthday parties held over the years, bringing with them all of the laughter, squabbles, heartaches and joys that accompany being a lucky member of a variety pack called family. The quiet was yet another reminder of fleeting time. I watched Billy knock billiard balls together on the pool table top, remembering his competitive spirit whenever he would partake in a game of eight ball with anyone willing to play. The table is rarely used now, the little ones are grown. Papa spends most of his days with Donna at their town house, and new traditions within the walls of separate family homes have replaced those once treasured at Grandma's house. Time marches on, and I reminded myself that the wise in spirit adjust accordingly and search endlessly and gratefully for joy in the *good ole days* at hand.

I sipped slowly on a hot cup of tea while taking in the view of the green rambling lawn before us, and the mighty Missouri River winding through a thicket of scarlet and gold. It eased that gratefulness in slowly. Billy held his warm cup in quiet contentment. I draped my arm over his shoulder, kissed him on the cheek and asked him if it felt good to be home. He nodded and patted my knee in approval. Our peaceful afternoon came to an abrupt end when one by one all of the hardworking residents of this beautiful place turned into the driveway and found their way home.

Clint and Lisa wasted no time in dropping by to visit and made plans for a fishing trip to Lake Frances on Saturday morning. The evening ended with a good dose of laughter, a belly full of warm dinner, and plans to tour our hometown beneath an umbrella of nostalgia the next day.

We were eager to cruise slowly from one memorable spot to another in the town where we had met, married, and shared the early years of our life together. The morning began with a few quiet moments, parked in front of the tiny little house Billy had purchased with hard-earned cash just as soon as he graduated from high school. It was a ramshackle house where he had spent many of those early years of wild abandon before he bumped into me. He let out a gasp and a "Hey!" when I turned the corner, pointing at the crooked front porch and the giant tree that had always shaded it. I took a deep

THE GREAT MOOSE'S TOUR

breath, secretly hoping he would remember.

"That's my house!" he finished.

He let out a sigh and his shoulders drooped as though he had instantaneously replayed each glorious memory in his mind. The relationships he built during those early years and the parties that little ramshackle house hosted were some of the finest days of his life and he spoke of them often. I watched the corner of his mouth turn up just a bit in a whimsical grin when we pulled away from the curb. I, too, held that place dear to my heart. I fell in love with Billy in there. It was Levi's first home, and the place where our young family tree took root. The sigh that escaped my lips was more bittersweet. I craved the power to turn the clock back to the time when Billy was young and his eyes glistened with adoration whenever I slipped into the front seat of his old blue Camaro in anticipation of another well-planned date that always left me feeling special. Time was my nemesis.

I pushed that sorrow down into the pit it rose out of and cheerfully asked Billy if he were up for a couple of greasy tacos from a local semi-Mexican restaurant. That particular restaurant had been termed *an acquired taste* over the years, and Billy and his brothers would joke about the necessary dining experience whenever any of them were in town. Before long we were facing each other from across a tall barroom table with a cold beer and a couple of Mexican-ish tacos topped with their house hot sauce that completed the dish. I helped Billy dollop the sauce on his tacos, wrapped them up tightly enough that he could maneuver them to his mouth and watched him savor every bite. He slowly rolled each swig of cold draft beer around on his tongue, and I was once again perplexed. He used to eat his meals so quickly and suck down a beer or two in no time flat, ready to get on to the next scheduled event. Now, it fascinated me, watching him so fully savor each bite, each sip, with calm enjoyment. If it hadn't been so confusing, I would have found it refreshing.

A quick trip through the quiet mall and a stop off at the grocery store found us on the back step once again licking our way through an ice cream bar and waiting for the family to arrive home from work that warm Friday night. The weather was perfect for a fire in Clint's backyard pit, and once chores and dinner were behind us, we cozied up next to the flames with a beer and a blanket and told jokes and old stories for hours. With a signaling yawn from Billy, Clint assured us that the boat was ready for one last fishing trip before winter set in and we headed for our cozy beds in anticipation of a full day on the lake.

Located on the outskirts of the little town of Valier, and a short drive north of Great Falls, Lake Frances is a small man-made reservoir stocked with plenty of perch, walleye, and pike. The short distance makes it an easy day trip for fishing, so after a leisurely breakfast and several cups of coffee, we loaded into Clint's suburban, looking forward to the good old Montana fishing trip that we had been missing out on since our move at summer's beginning. But the nearer we got to Valier, the skies of morning sunshine transitioned into a threatening bank of dark thunder clouds carried in on a chilly north wind, and although we all joked about the *walleye chop* the wind would provide on the surface of the lake, we were not looking forward to cinching up the hoods of our sweatshirts and fishing from beneath the protection of camping blankets Lisa routinely threw into the boat.

Montana fishermen are quite hardy, and a bit of chilly north wind hadn't deterred Clint in the least. While we were donning warmer gear, he began removing the cover and straps from the boat clad in just a t-shirt and his favorite BobCats ball cap. That cap symbolized his loyalty to the Montana State University football team he had been a member of for a short time during his glory days, and he never went fishing without it.

Not so long ago, Billy had been as hardy as any Montana outdoorsman, but recently, and with no apparent medical explanation, his body temperature was out of whack. And because he became chilled to the bone so quickly, I bundled him up first and poured him another warm cup of coffee from the thermos while we watched Clint back the boat into the choppy waters of the deserted lake. The walleye chop, rumored to stir up the silt from the bottom of the lake and jumpstart the fish's appetite, only gave Billy and me a nervous start to the day. Loading our lightweight boat back onto the trailer whenever we fished alone on Fresno Lake near our home in Havre had caused more than a few close calls with injuries. But Clint's strength and experience lent some relief as we climbed over the rails, scrambled under our blankets, and stowed ourselves next to the tackle boxes. The boat's motor lugged into a putter in defiance as we backed away from the shore, hoping to catch at least a few tasty perch and with any luck, a coveted walleye. The motor was still rebelling when Clint left his place at the helm and wobbled to the back of the rocking boat to diagnose its coughing and sputtering. Just as he reached the motor, it gave up and coughed a final puff of smoke and we sat idle in the water, thankful that we were not far from the dock. True to Clint's character, and not about to let the boat's motor dictate the day, he pulled its cover off and began to murmur under his breath while he tinkered with the intricate parts beneath. A few minutes of bobbing in the choppy water with the brisk wind threatening to blow us to an unsavory section of the bank, turned Clint's attention back to the trolling motor attached to the bow of the boat. The trolling motor was our ticket to an uneventful ride back to the dock and we were all silently hoping its battery had a strong enough charge to battle the wind that had become threateningly stronger. Clint was not able to find a quick fix for the motor and exasperation filled his face as he turned the boat into the wind. We puttered slowly back to the dock. With the disabled boat loaded safely back onto the trailer and our fishing trip cut short, we tucked our despondent and hypothermic bodies back into the warmth of the suburban for a sleepy ride home.

The chilly north wind was quickly left behind and we found much more pleasant weather awaiting us when the sunshine reappeared, warming our disappointment into determination to salvage the afternoon. Dinner plans, which would include Papa and Donna, quickly refueled the atmosphere. Papa and Donna had made it their routine to spend the work week at Donna's house in town and weekends at the family home in the country, and we found them puttering in the yard when we pulled in. Papa found humor in claiming to have two houses to call home, the *town house* and the *country house*. I, too, felt lucky for the privilege of being able to experience home in the extreme state of Montana as well as on the peaceful Oregon Coast, and reminded Billy of that gift often. Even in the midst of our daily unfolding tragedy, gratefulness at times became overwhelming and I found myself comparing our blessings of comfort and family to those less fortunate.

The barbeque was fired up early in the evening and soon an abundance of homegrown burger patties, grilled to perfection and dripping in melted cheese, were nestled amongst a variety of toppings and warmed buns waiting to adorn the mouthwatering morsels. Papa and Donna were ushered to a comfortable spot next to Clint at the dining room table and a hearty plate slipped in front of each of them. Papa and Clint were equally compassionate when it came to drawing Billy into the conversation, intermittently chuckling at his feeble attempt of storytelling and giving him a sense of comforting inclusion. Papa's rosy cheeks were a sign of his regained strength since his surgery not so long before, and sitting knee-to-knee with Billy, my fist holding up my weary head by one cheek, I was allowed the privilege of watching my aging father and my terminally ill sweetheart, share a fleeting moment in time. I watched in silent admiration and greedily observed these special men in my life, until that damn stomach knot reappeared and shocked me out of my euphoric state, instantly dissolving my bliss and harshly reminding me that these good ole days were in their final stretch.

Papa and Billy tired quickly, and after an hour or two of wine sipping and laughter, the twinkle in their eyes turned to squints and blinks signaling Donna and me to bid everyone goodnight and show our tired sweethearts to their beds.

All of Sunday was spent outdoors popping by each of my brothers' homes for short visits. They had been busy with winter preparations of cutting and splitting firewood and tidying up garden spots, but were happy to rest and catch up before we moseyed on to the next home, forcing them into a short break too. Nieces and nephews would cruise past on four-wheelers muffling the sound of chainsaws in the distance. The smell of the season filled the air, complete with the scent of sawdust filtering past the haphazard stacks of logs that had been trucked in from the mountains near Monarch.

My mind flashed back to the many fall weekends of our youth, riding in the rumbling old dump truck up the narrow and steep mountain road to Monarch where we would overstuff its rickety bed full of the logs dragged manually down the rugged hillsides. The smell of the Montana forests in fall is embedded in my memory and listening to the whir of the chainsaw and the smell of fresh cut pine was as comforting as the company shared in its midst. With late afternoon sunshine warming our shoulders and a crisp fall breeze tickling our cheeks, we plopped back down on the step at Papa's house with a contented sigh and contemplated our journey back to the beach the next morning.

It was now mid-September, and with each sunrise winter loomed larger on the horizon. The lawn we had planted was now a healthy runway of green, our freshly poured patio was ready for use, and the new hot tub was waiting for delivery. The Great Moose's Tour had come to an end and we were eager to put the finishing touches on our bubble.

We stopped only for fuel and potty breaks all the way to The Dalles where we stopped briefly to pick up Grandma Joyce, hoping to arrive in Lincoln City before nightfall. It was beginning to get dark much earlier in the evening and by the time we reached the VanDuzer Corridor it was as dark as the Oregon forest can be. Winding through the dark tunnel of the corridor gave the last leg of our journey an eerie feel and I found myself slowing to allow my eyes to focus clearly on any moving object that seemed to jump out at each turn. I was relieved when we finally popped out of the forest and into the well-lit streets of our new world.

Exhaustion consumed me when we pulled into the garage, realizing the burden of luggage, laundry, and mail that called for my immediate attention. Billy and Grandma Joyce had made their way into the house ahead of me, and when I finally stumbled into the kitchen lugging an armful of duffle bags, I found Billy sorting the stack of mail he had carried in and ripping much of it into bits before I had a chance to sort the junk from the pertinent pieces. My fatigue and frustration involuntarily spilled over, and his bewildered expression following my gruff lack of trust in his ability to do such a simple task as sort the mail nearly broke my heart. I dropped the bags where I stood, retrieved the balance of the untouched mail, and did my best to restore his confidence. The damage had been done, and he wandered out the front door and sat quietly on the porch chair while I finished unloading the rest of our trip's treasures from every nook and cranny of the car. Guilty tears stung my cheeks when, one by one, I began to wriggle all of the rugged sticks Billy had gathered, still covered with dried Montana mud, from the recesses of the trunk.

In a split second, I had made Billy feel he was a burden, and I vowed right then that I would never again be the cause of the disheartening fear that had furrowed his brow. I wiped away the tears, but the heaviness of guilt remained as I gathered the musty sticks and made my way to the front porch. Billy had focused his attention on the beams of light bouncing through the pine boughs from the nearby streetlight, but reached out his hand for one of his treasured sticks when our eyes met. Fear rarely made its way to Billy's outer surface, but I had awakened the realization that the monster was gaining ground and he looked to me for reassurance. I squeezed his hand tightly and apologized, hoping he would forget the entire incident by morning. He did.

Snuggling him tightly for a few minutes beneath the cozy blankets allowed time for the confusion of waking up in a different bed to wane. Jazzy wriggled out from under the covers he had tossed on top of her and began licking his face, causing a relaxed chuckle to escape and lighten the mood. The cloud of emotion I had taken to bed with me the night before had thankfully dissipated. But my heart ached with the truth. Billy's monster was now roaring from the shadows. Helplessness made me feel I was falling without a net most days, but I made a silent vow to never let my concerns affect Billy again and set out to make a healthy breakfast and a pot of coffee for him and Grandma Joyce. It was my birthday, and taking Billy and his mom out sightseeing in the Oregon sunshine was the gift I intended to give myself.

CHAPTER **13**

A BIRTHDAY TO REMEMBER

I FOUND BILLY and Grandma discussing world issues in a language all their own while nibbling at their breakfast and bouncing from one subject to another, complete with hand gestures and an air of comprehension. I was unable to gather their phrases into anything meaningful. I gave up and instead warmed their coffee and my heart by simply observing them sharing breakfast together in our home.

I silently watched. Would this be the last time Billy would share my birthday with me? How many last times had already floated by unnoticed? If it were my last birthday with Billy, I would spend it intentionally aware of his presence, his smile, his scent, and his gentle spirit.

It began with a trip to the local thrift store. Billy and his mom loved to hunt for treasures amongst trash and it soon became the theme of the day. Morning slid into afternoon by the time they had thoroughly investigated every shelf of every aisle and each had a few discoveries they couldn't pass up. Grandma beamed with delight, including Billy in the definition she proudly gave herself while we were carefully stowing their newfound treasures into the trunk.

"See Billy," she declared, "you and I, we're junkers!"

Billy shot me a grin, assuring me he remembered that Grandma had always been a collector of discarded treasures and a garage sale fanatic. I muffled a giggle and buckled him into his seat.

A stroll along the historic bayfront in Newport, followed by a birthday lunch at Mo's was next on the agenda, and slow-moving afternoon traffic allowed me to share in Billy's silent wonder of the drive and claim it as another little birthday gift. Pacific Highway 101 runs parallel to the coast, and the endless horizon melding into the intrigue of the beach far below the rugged sea cliffs is often in full view. I watched for the sign marking the turn-off to Devil's Punchbowl State Park, a well-known tourist attraction that the weather had often deterred us from experiencing on our previous trips to Newport. A gift of sunshine was inviting us on that particular afternoon. I leaned far over the guardrail to feel the salty spray from waves crashing in and swirling back out through the giant cauldron of sandstone known as the Devil's Punchbowl, adding one more unexpected snapshot into my growing scrapbook of adventures.

We found the Bayfront bathed in sunshine and tourists, and we merged effortlessly into the crowd, popping in and out of whatever shop caught Billy or Grandma's attention. My insides were all warm and fuzzy when we finally slid into a booth near the window at Mo's. The server handed us our menus and Grandma made several mentions of my birthday before we could finish with our orders. I leaned in close to Billy and asked him if he needed help deciding what to choose.

He adjusted his glasses, pulled them down, put them back up, cleared his throat and murmured,

"I'm, hahmmm, not sure."

I began pointing to several items on the menu, and with an exasperated sigh he finally agreed to a cheeseburger and a beer, his long-standing favorite. I wondered if his eyesight had been changing, or if he was no longer able to recognize the words he was trying so hard to read. Scheduling an appointment for an eye exam was tucked away in my mind.

I no longer felt quite so warm and fuzzy. I slipped my sweater over my shoulders and focused on including Grandma into the conversation while we enjoyed the lunch she was treating us to. Finally, our plates were cleared and several servers placed a slice of birthday cake topped with one lit candle in front of me and burst into song. Grandma's childlike excitement was worth every second of embarrassment that followed. Billy's laughter was infectious and Grandma's chest puffed up when she proudly snatched the bill and wriggled out of the booth on her way to the cashier. Birthday gifts popped up around every corner and I forced myself into continual acknowledgement of each one.

We sauntered slowly past the shops and back to the car with the warm afternoon sun caressing our shoulders. My mind was recounting the events of the day when I realized I had taken a wrong turn and noticed the sign marking the miles to Corvallis. I pulled into the next available turnout and heard Grandma let out a gasp. She had spotted a rundown shack in the distance, guarded by a field of thorny bushes dripping with ripened blackberries. While she grew more excited at the bounty of blackberries she was hoping to pick, Billy's attention went directly to the dilapidated building that was beckoning him to explore. I handed Grandma an old plastic container kept in the car for Jazzy's water and she went about tiptoeing through the thorny bushes and tall grass gathering the juicy purple gems. I followed Billy through the open door of the shack where the musty earth filled our nostrils and permeated throughout its one damp room. A strange faded pink sofa, its moldy foam spilling out from tattered edges, adorned one moss-covered wall and a rickety shelf of rusted canned goods was perched high on the opposite side. We could only assume from the contents that it had been a fishing shack at some point, and I urged Billy not to touch anything and follow me out. He continued to poke around and tugged open a rusty trap door on the outside of the building. I was cautioning him not to put his hand into the dark opening, but he reached in and pulled out a dusty handful of old dvds. He had caught Grandma's attention by then and she set her bowl, overflowing with berries, down in the tall grass and joined Billy in shaking the layers of dirt from the shiny treasures. Their excitement was hilarious and once again Grandma announced, "See Billy, we really are junkers!"

The semi-clean dvds were stowed next to the thrift store cache and the blackberries tucked safely on the floorboard in the back seat before we turned the car back in the right direction and started for Lincoln City.

We had just pulled into the parking lot of the grocery store, intending to pick up a few dinner items when my cell phone rang. Robyn's voice blurted out that he and Ryan had just lifted our new hot tub over the fence with a crane and onto the concrete patio. With excitement lighting up Billy's face, we rushed home to make sure they had set it down exactly where we had planned. It glistened in the sunshine, and with a scoot to the right and a shimmy to the left, it had found a permanent spot in our new backyard. Before long the tub was filled with icy water and we had been given instructions on how to balance the necessary chemicals throughout the winter months.

Our project was complete. Billy had a shiny new hot tub warming to perfection and waiting to soothe his body and spirit once we returned from taking Grandma back to her home in The Dalles. It was a perfect finish to a perfect birthday filled with discreetly revealed gifts.

CHAPTER **14**

HUNKERING DOWN

WITH OCTOBER NOW spilling over with the warmth that had eluded us throughout much of the summer months, siestas on the back porch became a favorite pastime. Nestled comfortably into our new reclining patio chairs with a crisp microbrew in our hands, a plate of smoked salmon and crackers between us, and the roar of the mighty Pacific rumbling in the distance, we escaped once more to our sun-drenched oasis. Our eyes met, and again the frequent and painful knot that had become a permanent tenant in the pit of my stomach forced me into resentful admission that the brilliance in the blue of my Billy's eyes had nearly disappeared. They seemed hauntingly vacant as he squinted and slowly closed them, resting his head back into the shade of the patio umbrella. Watching his chest rise and fall with the restful breaths of sleep, I pictured the monster's ravenous consumption of brain cells left weakened by the steady growth of protein-laden tangles, making it steadily more difficult for the electrical parts of his beautiful brain to function effectively.

It had also become far more noticeable by that time that Billy's speech had been reduced from broken sentences to bits of thoughts, and at times his expression could no longer hide the frustration he felt as he strained to transport single words past the fields of tangles to my patiently waiting ears. I had become neurotically over-protective of him and found myself shielding him from neighborhood acquaintances or store clerks in an attempt to protect him from the agony of difficult conversation and confused stares from those unaware of our ongoing war. So many roles in our relationship had been reversed.

I, too, closed my eyes against the bright sunlight and reminisced of all the times my husband had placed a protective hand at the small of my back as we entered a room, or the way he guided me to the inside of the sidewalk whenever we walked near traffic. He was no longer capable of opening the car door for me as he so often did, and it had become my responsibility to lead *him* into the passenger seat and assist him in buckling his seat belt. *I* had become the protector, dissolving one more brick from our partnership of marriage. I squinted away the pool of tears welling up behind my eyelids and begged The Giver for an extension of summer's joy.

That was a perfect fall day. I leaned over and kissed Billy on the cheek. He peered at me through sleepy eyes. I reminded him of the *Artoberfest,* and at the mention of handcrafted beer samples, he stretched his arms far above his head, let out a raspy yawn and zipped his Oregon Ducks pullover snugly up under his chin. He was ready to go. Our very significant summer had melted into a peaceful fall, and with the setting of the sun on that perfect fall evening came a growing awareness of so many last times nearly ready for harvest.

Fall gently slipped into winter and the rains eventually overpowered the sunshine for days at a time, forcing us to *hunker down* and wait them out. Billy spent most of the rainy days transforming his Montana sticks into works of art, while I converted a few into unusual, yet functioning bits of decor. Long walks through a misty drizzle whenever the heaviest of the rains relented became a prescription to relieve cabin fever and reminded us of the picturesque setting we were allowed to call home. We spent every waking moment together; cherishing life's routine and ending nearly every day with a good long soak beneath a foggy night sky in the steamy water of Billy's hot tub.

Billy continued a toddler's attempt at daily chores: making the bed, emptying the dishwasher, or taking Jazzy on long walks around the neighborhood. But within weeks, I began to find the comforter upside down and beneath the blankets, locating kitchen utensils became a scavenger hunt, and managing Jazzy's leash became a challenge for him. He didn't seem to notice, and I continued to encourage him with chores, fully aware that the monster's appetite was growing with each passing day. I concealed my concerns when he insisted he was capable of a short walk without me and I armed him with a walkie-talkie, hoping it would be possible for him to use it should he get disoriented. The days melted away and before we knew it the Thanksgiving holiday was upon us.

Billy was the oldest of his four brothers and two sisters, and that year was one of the rare occasions the four brothers would be gathered around the same dinner table. Autumn had finally landed a registered nursing job and was not able to join us, but Levi had a break from school and looked forward to a few days at the beach and Thanksgiving dinner with Jamie's family and his uncles.

One by one, family members arrived, and before long Jamie's home was brimming with holiday chaos. Molly and her parents were busy with traditional family recipes in the kitchen while Jamie added final touches to the table settings in the dining room. Rick, and his wife, Linda, were snuggled up on the sofa after their long flight, and Gregory, the youngest brother, had been popping in and out of the kitchen snitching bites and teasing his nieces about boys and fashion. Levi and I were assisting Jamie with details when my eye caught Grandma leaning over to generously refill Billy's wine glass, for what was undoubtedly the umpteenth time. I slid my hand between the bottle and the rim sending both Grandma and Billy into a full-blown pout. Billy had become far less tolerant to the effects of alcohol and I had been guarding his consumption like a hawk. But shortly after I showed him to his seat at the table and placed a full plate of Thanksgiving delights in front of him, it became obvious that I had not been vigilant enough. After a few feeble attempts at properly using his silverware, exhaustion consumed him and he let his fork fall into his dinner plate. His vacant stare and nauseated expression signaled me to remove him from the table and make him lie down. I left my dinner untouched and guided him slowly up the staircase with one arm under his elbow and the other firmly around his waist. It took much effort to twist his uncooperative limbs out of his clothes and wrangle him into bed, but the moment his head hit the pillow he began to snore. I slipped quietly back into my place at the dinner table next to the conspicuously empty chair beside me and silently prayed that the alcohol wouldn't bring about another *out-of-body experience* like the one I had witnessed earlier in the summer. A thankful heart carried me through the rest of the evening when I looked up to meet Levi's smiling eyes, and just a bit of my weariness faded when he whispered,

"I love you, Mom."

Dinner dishes were cleared promptly and while Billy slept, a traditional dice game ushered in another round of chaos and laughter. One by one the losers exited the game, a lucky winner gathered a bounty of dollar bills, and goodnight hugs were generously passed around. I slipped into bed next to Billy where he had been sleeping peacefully for hours, giving me one more reason to be thankful.

I awoke the next morning to a sense of urgency tugging at my spirit. I had been contemplating the possibility of a Hawaiian adventure while Billy was still physically able to participate, and with the previous evening's events etched into my mind, the trip's necessity had been confirmed.

With Billy's morning routine complete, I filled our coffee mugs and flipped open my laptop. Levi sat up from his slumbering position on the sofa behind me, and with his face twisted into a long yawn, attempted to ask what I was up to. Extravagant vacations were not Billy's style and we had always been content with our annual trips to the beaches of Oregon, so it was understandable when Levi squinted one eye and skeptically asked if I were teasing him.

An emphatic, "Nope! Not joking, Lovie," spurred him into action, and within seconds he had plopped down next to me. He joined me in wide-eyed excitement while we flipped through pictures of the resort on the island of Maui where Jamie and Molly suggested we stay.

We plotted, planned, and dreamed for several hours before agreeing on a tentative plan and calling Autumn to break the exciting news. Autumn let out a squeal of delight once we were able to convince her of the seriousness of our plan and was eager to share it with Kevin, her now very serious boyfriend.

We set the dates for late February when Levi had a final scheduled break from medical school, which also allowed Autumn the opportunity to schedule time off from her new job far in advance. And, although Billy happily agreed to my latest adventure, and put all of his trust in *my* decision-making, my current display of fiscal irresponsibility left me with a dose of anxiety topped off with a bit of guilt. But with my give-a-shit still broken beyond repair, I once again took up the reins of wild abandon and sternly reminded myself that the last times were popping up all around us. I had become desperately aware that regret would carry a far heftier price tag than our final scrapbook of wild abandon. Giddy excitement followed us back to our bubble where we dreamed of a tropical beach, and shared the majesty of the Pacific with Levi before we returned him to the airport.

Shifting his backpack into a comfortable position, he threw his shoulders back, blew me another kiss with a wink, and waved goodbye. A contented smile lit up his face when I smiled back from behind the windshield, and he turned and disappeared through the revolving glass doors. Usual tears that surfaced whenever he or Autumn turned to go were squelched. I knew that Christmas was right around the corner and they would both be back soon. More neatly wrapped gifts had been placed in the fields just ahead and the anticipated thrill in opening each one had quieted the incessant roar of Billy's monster, if only for a while.

CHAPTER **15**

WINTER'S JOY

THE FIRST DAYS of December ran together into a watercolor of violet and gray, the darkness camouflaging the transition of sunrise to sunset and blurring the lines between day and night. Discarded days filled only with mundane duties of life lay regrettably behind me and I searched in vain for ways to bring light into the darkness. Although I forced an outward glimmer, inside my mood hung as low and heavy as the clouds. The monster's heaving breath left its stench throughout the house, yet Billy remained upbeat and seemingly unaware of its constant presence. Even his recent hospital stay to undergo a colonoscopy, and the added diagnosis of colitis that followed had not dampened his cheerful demeanor.

Every morning we would lace up his tennis shoes for his twenty minute run on the treadmill, followed by an assisted shower and a full body warm up with the blow dryer. Goosebumps caused an involuntary shiver when I blew warm air up under his t-shirt, and the giggle that followed always coaxed a smile from my dreary interior. I stared long at him one morning, after the giggle had relaxed into a childish grin. The dull blue of his eyes gazed back, and once again a tsunami of guilt washed over me. I had no right to wallow in my longing of yesterday, and with a renewed defiance against the monster's threats, I slipped Billy's feet into his rain boots and his arms into his heavy winter slicker. I tightened the hood up snugly around his face. We would embrace the darkness, and I would find winter's joy.

Taken by surprise at The Artist's blend of deep gray and violet hues greeting us through a damp mist engulfing the vacant beach, I was forced to stand in silent awe and imagine memories recently forfeited by not having braved the darkness.

Billy and Jazzy had wandered ahead of me along the water's edge, the pounding winter surf forming mounds of snow-white foam that floated over the sand in the salty breeze and danced around their feet. Even in the darkest days, the majesty of the beach had the power to lull me into a grateful state of mind, and with it came the vision of gifts still waiting, unopened, in nearby fields. Those visions forced in a bit of the light that I had been struggling to find.

A few weeks later, watching Autumn first and Levi shortly after, step back through those revolving airport doors and into view from my place behind the windshield replaced any remaining gray in my spirit with the glittering hues of Christmas gold.

We found Jamie and Molly's home aglow with twinkle lights adorning a sophisticated tree in the dining room. In the family room a casual tree stood, hosting hand-made ornaments from years gone by. And Jamie pointed out his very own whimsical tree, with a monkey sporting a University of Oregon t-shirt perched snugly in its middle and surrounded by glistening "O"rnaments of bright green and yellow. Jamie is a loyal fan of the Oregon Ducks and proudly displays a vast collection of *Duck* themed treasures. We giggled while Molly opened a bottle of wine.

Billy loved Christmas, and I recalled the many times shortly after Halloween, that he would drag our well-worn imitation tree out of its storage bucket from the corner of the garage, plop it down on the living room floor, and with a promise void of intent express his willingness to help decorate. Most often, he would pour himself a glass of wine and put on Christmas music, watching from his corner of the sofa and wearing a blissful grin. That same tree had been trimmed in nostalgic glory before we left our bubble, and it sat patiently waiting for us to return and indulge in the pleasures of our first Christmas at the beach.

But Jamie had several pre-Christmas activities planned for us first, and the main attraction would be the Grottos Christmas Festival of Lights. The Grottos Festival of Lights is a serene display of spiritual symbols outlined in vibrantly colored lights amongst the generously decorated trees throughout the grounds. It was also host to a large Christmas chorus featuring many of the region's finest choirs. Grandma Joyce was especially looking forward to the spiritual experience of the Grotto during the Christmas season and we were excited to share it with her for the very first time. Billy's side of the family was rooted deeply in the Catholic faith, and although I had not claimed Billy's religion through marriage, the special tribute given to Mary, the Sorrowful Mother of Jesus, through the Grotto held significant meaning for me as well.

We followed behind a slow-moving crowd of on-lookers through a light drizzle of rain and a deep ebony forest aglow with a supernatural illumination. Pauses in silent wonder of lighted sculptures all around caused frequent stops on our way to the chapel. There we found warmth in familiar Christmas carols filling the air. It was a magical night, and snuggled up elbow-to-elbow with Billy, Levi and Autumn, and all of Jamie's family in the pew, I bowed my head in thankful prayer and allowed the lyrics of Christ's birth to sink deep into my soul.

I carried a mood of Christmas peace back to the beach with me and allowed Levi and Autumn's vibrant presence to refill our bubble with a youthful energy. Within minutes of plopping down the last of the luggage from the car, Levi had slipped into his swim trunks and headed out the back door toward the steaming hot tub. Billy was ecstatic at the idea of all of us soaking up the warm water together beneath a blanket of Christmas stars and we wasted no time in joining Levi in the bubbling water. Billy tipped his head back and closed his eyes while I became captivated by the conversation between our children. The few years they had spent out in the world matured them quickly and I puffed up with pride at the intelligent exchange of information bouncing effortlessly between them. They discussed the science behind the birth and death of the stars lighting up the sky above us, humanitarian issues of countries they had each visited, and complex medical conditions they had both studied and witnessed. I silently acknowledged the fact that they would forever be my life's greatest contribution to the world.

Our little Christmas tree twinkled at us through the window, catching Levi's attention and spurring him into an eagerness to pass out the meticulously wrapped gifts stacked haphazardly beneath it before the precious minutes of Christmas Eve had ticked away. For as long as Levi and Autumn could remember, Billy had traditionally sat at the base of the tree on Christmas Eve, examining each gift before handing it to the lucky recipient and insisting we all share in the eager anticipation of its revelation. For just a moment Levi allowed disappointment to dim the twinkle in his eyes when it was agreed that I would assume Billy's spot at the base of the tree that year. The generosity of Levi's spirit is matched by Autumn's thoughtfulness and the twinkle in their eyes was restored when one by one, Billy and I were proudly presented with each of their perfectly chosen gifts.

Billy's monster had jostled each of us into new positions within our little family, and just as I found myself forced into the role of Billy's protector and guardian, Levi and Autumn graciously stepped in as mine. The loving arms of their willing spirits wrapped tightly around me were the only Christmas gifts I needed.

The spirit of Christmas danced around us the next morning and followed us to the beach where abundant sunshine had finally replaced the heavy hues of misty gray. Winter's joy had found its place in my heart.

CHAPTER **16**

A CRABBY NEW YEAR

CHARGED WITH HOPE and a generous supply of sunshine, I ignored the monster's steady rumble, and turned my attention to a new year of wild abandon. The first would be a day of crabbing off the shore of the Siletz Bay.

Armed with three triangle crab traps, a bucket, a dozen chicken drumsticks, and a thermos of coffee, Billy and I worked our way through a crowd of beachcombers soaking up rare winter sunshine. Billy poked around in twisted piles of beach sticks while I baited each trap with a drumstick and readied the strings for a good toss over my head in hopes of landing them into the deepest water of the bay. Dungeness crab are sucked into the Oregon bays with the incoming tide and sucked quickly back out as the tide retreats leaving a designated window of time for luring the tasty crustaceans into the traps.

We had the good fortune of bumping into a local crabber named Steve on the foggy Siletz Pier a few weeks before, and he had patiently supplied us with step-by-step instructions for using crab traps. I went over the instructions carefully in my mind before I readied the first one, swung it in a wide circle far above my head, and watched it sail through the air and splash down into the dark water. I wrapped up the slack in the string, fastened the stake firmly into the sand and moved on to the remaining two traps. A peek over my shoulder found Billy visiting with another hopeful crabber a few yards down the beach; and once the traps were soaking on the sandy floor of the bay, I quickly slipped a protective arm under Billy's elbow and released him from the difficult exchange of small talk. The fellow crabber was kind and full of energy, and before long we had been introduced to the group of regular crabbers he belonged to. They continued to give us helpful hints throughout the afternoon and shared in our excitement when I finally pulled up a keeper. By the time the tide began to ripple back out to the mighty Pacific through the gate of the bay, we had several keepers in our bucket waiting to be boiled and cracked.

The opposite bank of the bay was home to a herd of sea lions that I had been watching while I tediously rolled up the tangled strings of each trap. One by one they had lifted their drowsy snouts and slid clumsily from their spots on the warm sand into the icy waters. The smoky scent of campfires began to float through the dusky air, and the final rays of the January sun transformed the remaining crabbers into dark silhouettes as we turned back for one final look from the parking lot.

A full day outdoors had left Billy chilled and sleepy and he was content to rest by the fireplace while I boiled up our bounty and tucked them securely into the refrigerator.

The most rewarding months to hunt for Dungeness crab are throughout the fall, winter, and spring. In fact, any month that contains the letter "R" because Dungeness crab molt and mate during the months between May and August, leaving them with less quality meat within their softer shells. We boasted our catch to Jamie, and with several "R" months of crab hunting just ahead, we began planning to put our skills to the test in Garibaldi Bay just as soon as schedules allowed.

February dragged in responsibilities that had been set aside during the holiday months. I'd been dreading our upcoming appointment with an attorney who had agreed to help us get our legal affairs in order. And although I had a durable power of attorney drawn up in Montana, I had been wisely advised to seek legal guidance to update it, as well as create our wills.

The attorney's brightly lit office was a stark contrast to the dreary day peering through the window, adding an extra eye-catching sparkle to the unpleasant words embossed in shiny black ink that boldly read "**Last Will and Testament**" on each of the professionally prepared packets she slid onto the desk in front of us. Documenting the final wishes of my Billy's life while knowing those wishes could soon be fulfilled sent an eerie shiver up my spine that shook my entire body. I struggled to catch my breath and steady the pen the soft-spoken attorney had handed me after verifying details between numerous pages. I signed where instructed and passed the pen off to Billy. He spun the pen between his fingers for a moment, tapped the point on the designated line, and gave me a questioning look. I nodded to go ahead, pointing once again to the designated signature line. Again, he fumbled with the pen and began a slow and rigid attempt at the signature he used to scribble without effort. He struggled through each of the pages with an unsteady hand and finally put the pen gently back down on the desk and leaned back into the leather armchair. His face held little expression while the compassionate attorney reassured him of the validity of his signature by adding the confirmation of a notary seal. It was finished. Our final ducks were all in a row. The attorney rose from her seat and shook Billy's hand. He attempted a feeble smile and turned his face toward mine. I had no weapons to conquer his fear, and retreated with a weak suggestion that we do something fun.

Billy sat in pensive silence all the way to Depoe Bay where I had hoped to brighten his mood with an early Valentine's Day lunch from a window seat overlooking the bay. He picked at his lunch and quietly sipped his brandy-laced coffee. Even the violent crashing of winter waves against the seawall below hadn't brought out the spark of wonder I had become used to witnessing. I coaxed a smile from him when I leaned across the table and asked for a Valentine's kiss.

He politely puckered up and kissed me gently on the lips before resuming his gaze at the roaring ocean through the smudged glass of the restaurant window. He rarely acknowledged the monster's presence, but it had snarled directly into his face that morning and was impossible to ignore.

CHAPTER 17

MAHALO MAUI

THE SPORADIC COOPERATION of Billy's short term memory allowed him to bury the monster's taunts in the shadows of the night and wake with little recollection of the previous day's terrors. I began to rely heavily on the fresh start carried in with each sunrise, dressing in an armor of determination and doing my best to deflect the monster's toxic darts away from our bubble.

It was nearly time to meet Autumn in Portland where we would board an airplane and spend six long hours together thirty thousand feet above the Pacific Ocean, stretching the boundaries of my comfort zone with wild abandon. Levi would be meeting us at the airport in Maui, and a tone of disbelief still rang in his voice when I gave him the time and date for their surfing lessons.

Details and excitement gently pushed me right up to the security gate, fumbling with both Billy and my IDs, shoes, belts and carry-on baggage. I allowed my sense of humor to drive that bus and exhaled deeply once we were all buckled safely into our seats. Autumn squeezed my hand during take-off and before long anxiety melted into quiet joy when Billy leaned his forehead against the tiny window to get a clear view of the glistening sea rippling between infinite horizons far below. I relaxed into his regained sense of wonder. The smooth flight allowed six hours in midair to pass quickly and Autumn squeezed my hand once again when she noticed me bracing hard against the landing. The loud whoosh, rocking and rumble came to an end at the gate and we were safely on the ground in Hawaii.

Our little family was charged with anticipation when Levi appeared and together we scrambled onto the shuttle toward our waiting rental car. Once inside the rental car office, we left Autumn to watch over Billy and the luggage while Levi and I chuckled our way through a long line of tourists also waiting to explore the island. For reasons still a mystery to me and Levi, the attendant suggested an upgrade from a sedan to a less roomy, but far sportier red convertible Mustang that sat in clear view from inside the shop window. A "hell yeah!" from Levi closed the deal. Levi shook the key at Autumn and pointed at the bright red jewel sparkling in the parking lot, and her jubilant shriek made the challenge of cramming our luggage into the trunk, and Billy's and my legs into the limited leg room of the back seat worth every bit of slight inconvenience. With Levi behind the wheel and a balmy wind whipping around our faces, we cruised slowly along the highway, hugging a mountainside on the right and the tropical beach of the Pacific Ocean on the left. We finally came to a stop beneath a large canopy marking the entrance to the Hanua Kai Resort in Kaanapali, our home for the next four magic-filled days.

A cool tropical breeze met us through an immense entrance unencumbered by the usual sliding glass door, allowing an expansive view of the Pacific just past the bustling and well-manicured grounds. Marble floors, glistening in every direction, led to a quaint coffee shop and several sitting areas complete with inviting patio furniture. A large decanter brimming with sparkling iced water and fluorescent slices of lemon and lime caught Autumn's attention and she slipped away to fill a complimentary glass. A brightly colored porcelain pot housing a vibrant and proud Bird of Paradise welcomed me to the front desk where I retrieved the key to our getaway and a permit for the parking garage below. I found Levi pointing out several large fish to Billy in a pond separating the lobby from the grounds. I handed him one of the room keys before we strolled back out of the lobby.

Levi pulled the car into a well-lit spot in the garage and stowed the parking permit in the windshield. He and Autumn wriggled the luggage out of the car and nodded for us to follow them into the building, chatting and laughing the entire time. They had stepped in again as protector and guardian without giving it a second thought. Relief consumed me. I locked elbows with my Billy, a warm breeze caressing my body and soul, and followed Levi and Autumn through the squeaky door of the parking garage and into the sun-drenched hall leading to the elevators.

Our ninth floor view faced an emerald mountain, its summit encircled by an opaque cloud ring and crowned with a rainbow tiara. While duffle bags and suitcases exploded in search of beach attire, Billy flung open the patio door and a warm wind flooded the room with the mountain's royal beauty. It was late afternoon, and still hoping to soak up an hour or two of sunshine while sipping a tropical beverage from the comfort of a chaise lounge, we donned our suits, passed out beach towels and went in search of a perfect spot beneath the waving palm trees near the pool. Levi was quick to offer himself up as cocktail server, and with credit card in hand, he disappeared into Dukes restaurant in search of the bartender. Lava Flows and Mai Tais were passed around and before long we were melting into our surroundings, the gentle surf brushing the seashore and blending in perfect harmony with the orchestra of palm trees rustling in the steady breeze above our sleepy heads.

A good dose of Maui had been absorbed through our skin when the sun's warm glow dipped into our first Hawaiian sunset, and we wasted no time freshening up and making our way back down to an outdoor table at Dukes beachside restaurant for dinner.

Dukes, which honors Duke Kahanamoku, a Kanaka Maoli competition swimmer and the father of modern day surfing, also boasts a mesmerizing view of the Pacific laced with the islands of Molokai and Lanai. Captivated by the sunset's brilliance reflected on the surface of the water, we were startled when the hostess let out a gasp, and with an excited gesture forced our gaze to a rippling section of the water in the distance. We squinted against the sunset's glow just as several massive humpback whales breached out of the water and slapped their giant tails on the way back down.

Great humpback whales migrate from feeding grounds in Alaska to the warm waters of Hawaii for mating season each year, making Hawaii a popular whale-watching destination during the months of February and March. They are also more active during mating season, making breaching and tail slaps on the surface of the water more frequent. We were awestruck, staring along with many other diners and wait staff, waiting in vain for another incredible show. But there was no encore and the restaurant soon fell silent. Everything we ordered and shared had a surreal and tantalizing flavor. The evening breeze chilled us into a tight cluster under the patio umbrella and drew the four of us even closer into another precious snapshot of time.

With no time to waste, the morning's agenda held the task of acquiring the necessary equipment and instructions for a snorkeling adventure and we found our way to Snorkel Bobs near Napili Bay. By mid-morning we had each been fitted with a snorkel mask and breathing tube, as well as flippers and all of the guidance necessary for a safe and rewarding experience.

Also near Napili Bay was the highly recommended Plantation House, and with Levi's appetite begging for attention before our snorkel workout, we indulged in a sophisticated brunch overlooking the Plantation Golf Course. The ocean breeze, as well as a bird or two, blew freely through the historic floor-to-ceiling windows that opened up onto a rolling course of green velvet on one side and panoramic views of the Pacific on the other. Billy had been quiet most of the morning, but wore a cloak of contentment and relaxed against the chair back, slowly sipping coffee from an elegant china cup. The music of Levi and Autumn's laughter suddenly rang through the air when Levi shared a text message from a friend suggesting that he "Brunch hard!" and his insistent reply that we were, in fact, "Brunching hard!" at the Plantation House, on the island of Maui, in Hawaii. A constant air of pure bliss bubbled around Levi and Autumn everywhere we went and I held on tightly to Billy, snatching up the happy bits left in their wake.

Full bellies and a trunkful of snorkeling gear fueled a burst of nervous energy that led us to the crowded beach of Napili Bay an hour later. Levi patiently strapped Billy's fins over his feet, snugly fit his mask over his eyes and nose and repeated breathing instructions several times before we all tripped clumsily over our finned feet through the loose sand and down to the water's edge. Levi and Autumn waded into deeper waters ahead of me and Billy. I held tightly onto Billy's hand and we inched our way into the shallow water behind them. We shared an unsure look and with a jolt of bravery slipped under the water. We held hands and faced each other through the rocking waves, frantically sucking air from the tube above the surface. We struggled for a few minutes before we relaxed and looked to the busy floor of the bay, in curious appreciation of the underwater world we had imposed upon. Schools of neon-striped fish darted in and out of the abundant coral formations, and colorful sea plants performed a hula dance from their homes on moss-covered sea rocks. Suddenly, Billy pulled away and I popped my head above the surface to find him struggling with his mask and doing his best to tread water. It quickly became obvious that what I thought was confusion about clearing the water from his mask, was actually a state of panic and fear of drowning. We were not far from shore so I grasped his elbow and paddled with him to shallow water where we were able to stand. The spark that had once ignited my Billy's bonfire of youthful thrills had been snuffed out, and once his face was cleared of saltwater and fear, he was perfectly content to spend the remainder of the afternoon settled into a warm spot on the crowded beach.

For the next few hours, I stayed within eyesight of Billy while Levi and Autumn bobbed up and down in the deeper water hoping to catch a glimpse of a green sea turtle. One after the other they finally stumbled out of the water, worn out from their undersea exploration and disappointed that a sea turtle had not come out of hiding. They stripped the flippers from their shriveled feet and flopped down onto the warm blanket, hoping the afternoon sun still had the power to warm them. The sand covering their drenched bodies dried quickly, and brushed off easily when we stood to give the blankets a good shake before we started the long trek back to the sporty red Mustang and then to a much-needed shower.

We each emerged from the bathroom covered in a different hue of scarlet, which deepened as the evening wore on, and Aloe Vera oil was generously slathered all over our parched skin before we dressed for dinner.

The wind had blown much harder all day, and by the time we sat down for another outdoor dinner at Dukes, it was blowing a damp breeze throughout the candlelit dining area. Without reservations, sitting inside was impossible, and because the drizzle of rain delivered with our dinner had turned our sunburned chill into an uncomfortable shiver, we were forced to snuggle up even closer under the patio umbrella. We savored every bite as quickly as possible, eager to soak in the hot tub steaming nearby.

Tiptoeing into the hot water while allowing the tingle of our sunburns to wane was worth the soothing warmth of the steaming water against chilled muscles, and we soaked in the quiet comfort of each other's presence. I stared at the heavens, slid up next to Billy's side and relaxed into the whispering symphony of swooshing palm trees against a sky of midnight blue.

We rubbed our eyes against the early morning light when Levi and Autumn's cell phone alarms rattled the stillness. Surfing lessons in Lahaina began promptly at seven, and there was little time to slather on a much-needed dose of protective sunscreen before we slipped back into the Mustang, in search of the Maui Wave Riders surfing school. Once inside the quintessential surf shop, drenched in a casual atmosphere and bustling with instructors dressed in board shorts, Levi and Autumn were swept away and fitted with wet suits and a giant surf board. The experience had already become delightful when we followed Levi and Autumn out of the shop and down the narrow side streets of Lahaina lugging their cumbersome boards, with their energetic instructor leading the way. A few blocks later we tripped past an old warehouse and popped out onto a stretch of sandy beach. After a short lesson on balancing techniques in the soft sand, the instructor helped them onto their boards and paddled his way ahead of them beyond the rolling surf. From our shady resting spot on a brick wall beneath a twisted tropical tree, we watched the instructor shout and wave as they each attempted an upright position on their boards. Several tries later, they had each proudly ridden a wave back to shore in a full upright position, and for the next two hours they continued to paddle back out over the surf, clumsily regain their balance, and ride wave after wave back in.

By the time they dragged their heavy boards and bodies over the sand and dropped near our feet, they were exhausted. A few moments of rest allowed them to muster up their last bit of strength, struggle to their feet and lug the bulky boards back to the shop where they stripped off the wet suits, rinsed the remaining sand from their feet and sank onto a bench where we waited for captured memories to print.

They had worked up a hunger, and with plans to explore the quaint town of Lahaina, we wandered down the narrow streets in the opposite direction of the surf shop in search of a cheeseburger and an afternoon of souvenir shopping. Full bellies fueled a burst of energy a short time later, and while they were teasing each other about mishaps during the adventure and moaning about stiff muscles, Autumn spotted the Local Boys shaved ice shop. A tourist must, we each emerged with a full cup of multi-flavored ice mixed with sweet cream, and crossed the street to admire the famous Banyan Tree of Lahaina.

The tree was only eight feet tall when it arrived from India in 1873 and was planted near the courthouse by Sheriff William Owen Smith of Old Lahaina Town. Now standing fifty feet tall and a quarter mile around, it is anchored to the ground by over ten trunks giving the single tree an illusion of many trees. The Banyan tree grows by soil-seeking roots that hang down together until there are enough of them to form a strong trunk. Billy's sense of wonder was in overdrive while we slurped our creamy confection and strolled in bewilderment amongst the twisted trunks holding up the mystical behemoth.

When we finally stepped from beneath its shadows and back onto the sunny sidewalk, Autumn licked the last drop of creamy ice from her plastic spoon, tossed her empty cup into the trash and squeaked out a desperate plea to spend the remainder of the afternoon soothing her sore bones in the warm sunshine next to the pool. Not much convincing was required and another round of tropical drinks soon lulled us into an afternoon siesta beneath another brilliant Hawaiian sky crowded with dancing palm trees.

With a desire to fulfill Levi's request for a highly recommended breakfast of macadamia nut pancakes the next morning, another choir of alarms rustled us into action. The tiny Gazebo restaurant in Napili does not accept reservations, requiring hungry diners to arrive early in hopes of securing a place at the front of the long, winding line that forms outside of its door each morning. There was an exasperating line of chattering guests ahead of us when we finally fell in at the rear, leaving us to wonder if they had watched the sunrise from their spots in line. Boredom set in quickly and Autumn wandered off, camera in hand, to clamber over the beach rocks below the restaurant and explore the exposed tide pools. She returned just as we rounded the corner of the building and several hopeful diners began pointing far out to the water in front of us. We watched in awe as once again several giant whales breached their massive bodies out of the water, flopped back down with a thud and slapped their tails loudly on the surface before they disappeared. The encore we had not received during dinner at Dukes had become a circus of activity that brought life into the still waters of the early morning.

Boredom, along with the line, dissipated during the excitement and soon we were staring directly into a gigantic stack of fluffy white pancakes smothered in coconut syrup and topped with a generous sprinkling of fresh macadamia nuts and whipped cream. The velvety pancakes melted into the coconut sweetness of the syrup with each bite, and suddenly waiting in a line for more than an hour outside no longer seemed quite so silly. Leaning back in a lethargic stupor, we finished the decadent experience with a freshly brewed cup of Hawaiian coffee, unconcerned with the hustle and bustle of the compact and chaotic world swirling around us. We stretched, yawned, patted our bellies and sauntered back to the parking lot with rays of morning sunlight gently caressing our sunburned shoulders. We were ready for another full day of snorkeling adventures.

The best snorkeling in Mokuleia Bay is in the morning if the waves are calm, and because it was a short drive north of Kaanapali, it was first on our list. Hoping for calm waters and another chance at spotting a green turtle, Levi squeezed the Mustang into one of the few narrow spots that tightly hugged the guarded edge of a steep embankment to the front and whizzing highway traffic to the rear. In single file, we gripped the hand rail and cautiously made our way down a steep staircase carved into the earth and nearly hidden from view at its entrance. The final step popped us out from under the trees and onto a wide stretch of sparkling white sand, known as Slaughterhouse Beach. An old slaughterhouse, torn down in the mid-sixties, had long sat right at the edge of the sea cliffs above, giving the beach its unusual name.

Huge waves crashing onto shore greeted us and immediately dashed any hope of snorkeling in the dangerous surf. But it did not deter us from spreading out our beach blankets on the warm white sand and partaking in a wrestling match with the waves. Autumn followed Levi, Billy followed Autumn, and I followed Billy cautiously into the chilly waters of the taunting surf. Levi bounced his way out past a few larger waves and body-surfed his way back in, giving Autumn a false sense of confidence that she too could conquer a wave. Her tiny frame was quickly overcome by rushing sea water and with a gulp of fresh air, a frantic search for her swim top was immediately underway when she realized the triumphant wave had retreated with a souvenir. Levi arose victorious through the foamy waves with the tiny top in his fist and instantly became Autumn's knight in shining armor. We collapsed, laughing and exhausted onto the warm blankets, but soon fell silent, exhaling salty air and inhaling the warm bliss of yet another fleeting moment that would forever connect our hearts.

A short rest rallied us into action with a plan to snorkel Black Rock at Kaanapali Beach. The Sheraton Hotel near Whaler's Village allows access to the bay, and once the challenge of parking had been mastered, we strolled through the hotel grounds, weaving our way through a field of lounging guests until we reached the slender strip of sand bordering the bay. We squeezed our way into one of the few open spots on the sand and geared up. Levi and Autumn stayed in view for a few minutes before disappearing amongst the multi-colored swim bottoms bobbing to and fro like wildflowers in a field of waves. I stayed with Billy, listening to the hum of vacationers and watching for a familiar wildflower to pop up out of the water. It wasn't long before one did, wide-eyed and ecstatic at what she had experienced. We took turns exploring the calm waters around the jagged black lava rock, soaking up the sun with Billy for a little while before unanimously agreeing to leave the crowded beach and venture down to Mile Marker Fourteen.

Mile Marker Fourteen is located just off the highway with little parking or beach, but was recommended by locals as a rewarding experience for beginners. Levi managed to maneuver the Mustang off of the busy highway and nestle it safely beneath a gnarly beach tree not far from the water's edge. Billy and I were far less interested in the world beneath the sea by that time and snuggled up on a blanket together while Levi and Autumn went in search of the elusive green turtle. Once again, I peered over the water's shining surface hoping to keep an eye on the hot pink bottom of Autumn's suit. We blinked and she disappeared into a sea of snorkelers, leaving us to wait and hope that there wasn't a shark lurking nearby. Levi would give me an exasperated sigh whenever I warned of the possibility of sharks, and did little to tame a display of frustration when he tripped out of the water in a frenzy, certain something terrible had happened, only to discover that I had been waving my arms frantically in the fear that he had ventured out too far.

Autumn had already joined Billy and me on the blanket by then after a claustrophobic experience not long after she followed Levi into the surf. Mountains of coral sat just beneath the surface of the shallow water, creating valleys between them deep enough for Autumn to snorkel through but not deep enough to float over. A maze of sharp coral had trapped her and she was unable to safely turn herself around. She floated in the valleys of coral until a large wave washed over her, allowing her to crest the sharp peaks of the coral and swim to shore. Frightened to give it a second try, she stretched out in trembling relief next to her daddy and let the warm sun melt away the fear.

Levi shot me a *don't do that again* glare before he slipped back under the water and out of sight. We waited patiently on the tiny beach, littered with sharp twigs and rocks, hoping he would emerge safely, all the while envisioning a tropical beverage and a lounge chair nestled safely by the pool. Finally, he popped up, clearing seawater from his mask and sputtering colorful descriptions of all the grand sea life he had encountered. Although Autumn and I were ready to leave Mile Marker Number Fourteen in the rear view mirror forever, it was impossible to be annoyed that Levi had been gone so long when the excitement from his enchanting underworld adventure continued to spill over all three of us.

A rest by the pool, a soak in the hot tub, and a delicious dinner left us dripping with contentment. Another magical sunset glistened on the water and a warm breeze tickled our cheeks while we strolled side-by-side over the sandy bluff to the beach. Levi turned to me, his handsome face lit up with joy, and pointed out to the sunset's shimmering glow illuminating the heavens and lighting up the ocean with dancing twinkle lights.

He waded out to his knees, captivated by the grandeur before him, unwittingly filling me with pride. Billy, Autumn, and I stood in silence, caressed in peace, watching Levi up to his knees in the Pacific Ocean, baptized in The Artist's brilliant glory. The monster was nowhere to be found on that final evening in Maui.

The mountain outside of our window watched proudly from beneath her rainbow tiara while we stuffed our island treasures and

Chapter 6

52. Tina Peters, interview with the author, September 23, 2016.
53. Ibid.
54. Ibid.
55. Ibid.
56. "Sustainability," Fort Collins Brewery, accessed October 2016, http://fortcollinsbrewery.com/sustainability.
57. Peters, interview.
58. Ibid.
59. "Fort Collins Brewery Releases Limited-Edition Oud Bruin," Brewbound.com, accessed October 2016, http://www.brewbound.com/news/fort-collins-brewery-releases-limited-edition-oud-bruin.
60. "About," FOCO Café, accessed October 2016, http://fococafe.org/about.
61. Peters, interview.
62. Ibid.

Chapter 7

63. "About Us," Funkwerks, accessed September 2016, http://funkwerks.com/pages/about-us.
64. Brad Lincoln, interview with the author, September 16, 2016.
65. "Great American Beer Festival 2012 Award Winners," accessed November 2016, https://www.greatamericanbeerfestival.com/wp-content/uploads/12_GABF_winners.pdf.
66. Lincoln, interview.
67. "About Us," Horse & Dragon Brewing, accessed September 2016, http://www.horseanddragonbrewing.com/who-is-horse--dragon.html.
68. Carol Cochran, interview with the author, September 23, 2016.
69. Ibid.
70. "Sustainability," Horse & Dragon Brewing, accessed October 2016, http://www.horseanddragonbrewing.com/sustainability.html.
71. "Events," Horse & Dragon, accessed September 2016, http://www.horseanddragonbrewing.com/hd-half-marathon--pint-run.html.
72. Kirk Lombardi, interview with the author, September 16, 2016.
73. "About," Zwei Brewing, accessed November 2016, http://zweibrewing.com/about.aspx.

dirty laundry back into our duffel bags the next morning. The Giver had given another precious last time, a window of time, just the four of us. Time. Grasping for precious time had forever untethered me from the constantly moving world.

We prepared for departure and waited once more outside of the Gazebo restaurant in the morning sunshine. We couldn't help ourselves—one final immersion in touristy chaos. It was right next to Napili Bay after all, and we had hours before our flights. We waited in the line, peered out to the sparkling waters in hopes of another whale-watching extravaganza, and indulged in breakfast delights. With another belly full of sweet pancakes, we went in search one final time for the elusive green turtle. Billy still had no interest in a second attempt at the breathing tube, so Levi, Autumn, and I took quick turns scouting the underbelly of the bay while he waited patiently amongst a sea of fellow sunbathers.

I was looking for Autumn's bathing suit bottom again when they both popped up, waving ecstatically. They had spotted one! A big green turtle had wiggled out of its hiding spot behind a giant rock and floated just beneath them. After snapping a few photos with the underwater camera, Levi sat with Billy while Autumn and I snorkeled back out. Just as soon as I dipped my mask below the water, I, too, had the joy of observing the elusive green turtle paddling nonchalantly beneath me in the murky waters of Napili Bay. It was a perfect finish to our Maui adventure.

We parted ways with Levi at the airport. He would take Hawaiian Air back to Phoenix. We would fly Alaskan into Portland. I watched him stroll away, shoulders back, chin up, his wavy hair lightened by the tropical sun. He turned, as he always does, waved and blew me a kiss attached to a wink. He was gone. Another last time.

Most of the way home, we held tightly to each other through the worst turbulence the flight attendant had ever experienced, leaving us relieved that our final extravagant adventure, filled with days of wild abandon had come to a safe end, and we would soon be nestled back into our bubble at the beach. Home, with my Billy.

CHAPTER 18

GLORIOUS GARIBALDI

WHILE WINTER'S GRIP weakened, the monster's grip grew stronger. It had been stealthy, quietly snatching bits of Billy while we were busy. The challenging game of communication had left a desperate plea in Billy's eyes. I searched hard past the dull blue of his stare. He was in there. My Billy was in there, trapped between the tangles, claustrophobic, and fighting to be heard. I vowed to listen, not with my ears, but with my heart. I watched for signals in his eyes, the mirrors of his soul. I wanted him to *feel* me listening.

I looked ahead to the energy of spring. A lighthearted atmosphere blew in with Rick and Linda when a school break allowed them to visit with his daughter, and Jamie and Molly refilled our bubble with enthusiasm when they ushered Rick's family through our front door and immediately rallied everyone into action. A whirlwind of beach activities left us dizzy a short twenty-four hours later when the door closed behind them. They were gone as quickly as they came.

Silence, more deafening silence. But when I glanced at Billy, his face was glowing, his eyes were smiling. Billy and Rick had been warriors together through battles of a dark youth, and victory had locked their scarred spirits together. Rick's visit had sparked a happy light. Spring had sprung.

Rick's uplifting visit led directly into our long awaited crabbing trip to Garibaldi Bay. Billy bustled around, picking things up, putting things down, sweeping random bits around in the garage the evening Jamie arrived to ready the boat for our adventure. The bright lights of the garage bounced back against the ebony of the forest, illuminating our corner of the block. Jamie rigged each crab pot in the chilly evening air, charged the boat's batteries, and stowed our raingear into the pickup.

We were up with the sunrise and before long lunch was packed, a thermos was filled to the brim with steaming coffee, and the boat was securely hitched to the pickup. A final check of the tide table and we were ready. Low tide would be midday, allowing plenty of time for the scenic two-hour drive north on Highway 101. The sounds and smells of the rolling surf, mixed with the musty dampness rising up from the forest floor, floated in through my nostrils and infused my fibers. I snuggled up next to Billy in the cozy cab of the pickup, relaxed against his shoulder and wove my fingers into his. Crashing waves popped in and out of view through the windshield and I squeezed my eyes shut in another feeble attempt to slow time.

Jamie broke the mood when Garibaldi Bay caught his eye and he began to giggle. It was nearly ebb tide, and the mighty source of the bay was still sucking water through its gateway and taking all the crab with it. We had arrived far too early. Our eagerness was cause for a steady round of laughter when we finally pulled into the parking lot.

With time to kill before the crab would be washed back into the bay with the incoming tide, we bellied up to the bar of the Troller Lounge on Fisherman's Wharf for a mid-morning beer and French fries. Jamie and I shared the same love of the seventies music and décor as Billy did, and the Troller Lounge had remained comfortably suspended in that decade. The seating area was smattered in hues of deep orange and olive green amongst an abundance of wood paneling. And with Billy between us, we plopped down on a bar stool and reveled in the time warp we had stumbled upon, still giggling at our arrival long before the crab.

When we noticed the bay beginning to fill a bit, Jamie carefully backed the boat into the water. He stowed the pickup safely in the lot, lumbered down the dock in his bulky rain boots, stepped over the rail and slid in behind the wheel. I tucked Billy safely into the seat next to the captain's chair and watched in quiet admiration as Jamie's gentle eagerness replaced Billy as captain of the boat. Billy's body relaxed, his arm draped over the side of the boat, and a wondrous gaze bounced from seagull to seagull as they screeched above us on our way out to deeper waters. Moments of joy were the weapons making up the arsenal with which I continued to battle back the monster, and Jamie had become my comrade in arms.

Jamie and I agreed that we must have both been deep sea fishermen in a previous life, although very little expertise carried over to the present. Jamie often mimicked George Clooney's character from the movie *The Perfect Storm*, holding up a fist and declaring "I always find the crab!" and Molly quickly dubbed him *Captain George* whenever he stepped onto the boat. He wore the title proudly as he stood at the helm, one knee on the seat behind him, one hand on the wheel, and the other pointing ahead to fertile waters in which to drop our pots. I did my best to be a helpful deckhand, wrapping line and throwing in pots at his command. For several hours, we mingled between seasoned crabbers and floated through an obstacle course of buoys attached to pots at the bottom of the bay. Billy's laughter warmed the air when tiny crab escaped the confines of each pot we pulled up and scurried around the bottom of the boat. We continued to pull pots and sort crab until we were one of the few boats left on the bay. By the time the tide began to recede we had eighteen keepers bouncing around in the live well. Captain George was thrilled at our catch and the success of our first Garibaldi excursion. We replayed the events of the day all the way home and were eager to include Molly and Maddy in our next adventure.

CHAPTER 19

MAYHEM IN MAY

MAY'S ARRIVAL WAS drenched in sunshine and damp heat that drew us outside nearly every day. We were busied with yardwork and the thrill of mowing our tiny stretch of healthy new lawn, trimming and weeding plants requiring attention, or planting new ones chosen by Billy with the help of a vendor at the Farmers Market. The wheels of wedding planning had also been set into motion once Kevin finally called and requested our permission for Autumn's hand in marriage. We danced in our delusion of normalcy to the music of long walks through the forest or combing the beach for treasures, finishing most afternoons with our routine siestas beneath the shade of the patio umbrella.

Weeks of uneventful bliss, along with our illusion of safety, were shattered late one afternoon while Billy sat quietly at the kitchen counter watching me repair a leaky faucet. I glanced up just in time to witness his shoulders droop, his eyes roll back and his head fall forward. He quickly sat back up, visibly shaken and pale, but before I could lay him down on the couch behind us, his color had returned and he was wondering what had happened. Fearing I may have witnessed a mild heart attack, I slipped on our shoes and jackets and went straight to the emergency room.

Several hours and numerous tests later, we were released with no explanation. No indication of a heart attack was found, but with the possibility of an abnormal heart rhythm, we were sent home with a monitor strapped to his waist in hopes of catching the pesky arrhythmia.

Forty-eight hours later, no sign of an arrhythmia left us with another shrug of the doctor's shoulders, and the confounding explanation that this monster's behavior is often unpredictable. I was on guard, anxiety riddled my daily routine, and Billy was never far from my sight. The monster had taken full advantage of my previous state of bliss; and, refusing to be ignored, had snuck a dart past my armor and left our precious bubble with a slow and steady leak.

The next weeks were spent in constant vigilance. I obsessed over his pallor, his breathing, his gait. I listened while he slept, laying my head on his warm chest fearfully waiting for an interruption in the symphony that kept my Billy here in the physical world with me. The orchestra played on, Billy maneuvered through each day in a child-like state of apathy, seemingly unaware of my obsession. I fell back into a more guarded version of our routine, fully aware that the monster had become a formidable opponent, yet unwilling to yield to his inevitable victory without a good fight.

With Billy's strange episode appearing to have been random and singular, we settled into our backyard oasis on a sunny June afternoon to begin plans for the second annual Moose's Tour. Billy squinted uncomfortably through the bright rays of the afternoon sun, and when he stood to slide his chair into the shade, I stood too, reaching up to open the patio umbrella. But before I could manage to secure it, I heard Billy trip and fall into the lounge chair behind me. I turned to find him twisted and tangled into the chair, not moving, his blue eyes wide open, dull and lifeless. Panic took the wheel. I shook him hard, screaming for him to wake up. The chaos of my fear only grew when Billy suddenly shot each arm out to the side and his entire body became rigid, quivering as though he had touched a livewire. Within seconds, it was over. His body relaxed, his spirit reappeared into the weary blue pools of his eyes, and I cried. He was confused. He didn't understand my tears. I struggled to get us both to our feet and into the house where I convinced Billy to rest while I composed myself and called Dr. O.

Dr. O. scheduled another round of tests and requested that we put the second annual Moose's Tour on hold while precious weeks of summer were spent in search of an elusive cause to Billy's loss of consciousness. A measure of seizure activity in his brain, an ultrasound of his aorta, a month of recording heart rhythms, and a cardio stress test left us with instructions to monitor his blood pressure for serious drops, followed by another *wait and see* response.

A much needed reprieve from the stresses of summer's beginning arrived with Billy's sister, Tammy, during a summertime adventure with her son, Kayden. Billy had earned a trusted spot deep in Tammy's heart when he stepped in as silent hero, offering an unconditional refuge from an unrelenting storm in her younger years. Although their bond was not discussed, it remained, and her need to share time with Billy held great personal importance.

Tammy's intrepid and adventurous spirit had always intrigued me, and spending the Fourth of July holiday with her and Kayden left me hoping to refresh the stale air pressing against our bubble's weakened shell with the positive light swirling freely around her. Her non-intrusive personality slipped in quietly and immediately lifted our moods. She allowed Kayden to shop in excited anticipation within the temporary walls of a local fireworks tent before we trudged together through the chilly evening wind and blowing sand to huddle beneath blankets on the beach, where he entertained us with an amateur fireworks show. The entertainment ended abruptly, however, when poor Kayden was frightened into submission by a beach patrol officer who put a stop to the forbidden thrill. We giggled all the way home and finished up the colorful display from the comfort of the garage, where drops of fluorescent brilliance bounced against the darkened backdrop of the forest and warmed the evening air, along with our laughter into the wee hours.

CHAPTER **20**

THE NOT-SO-GREAT "NO" MOOSE'S TOUR

FOURTH OF JULY'S sparkle faded, along with Tammy's air of joy when we reluctantly waved goodbye the following morning and reality squeezed its way back in. Billy was slowing down. His breathing had changed. He puffed a bit when we strolled to the far end of the beach when the tide was low. He napped more. With a heightened awareness of the content of every single moment, I intentionally slowed life's pace, taking in his presence and always wondering how many more moments The Giver would allow.

Dr. O. did not recommend a long road trip back to Montana that summer, but with no concrete medical reason that it should be unsafe and my promise to stop and stretch Billy's legs frequently, he finally gave his guarded approval to go ahead with the second annual Moose's Tour. But because apprehension did not allow for the journey further north to Moose's Saloon, visiting *home* became our theme and arriving there without incident our journey's only goal.

Billy slid contentedly into his seat on a warm August morning, grinning as I buckled him in for the second annual, Not-So-Great *No* Moose's Tour. I stowed last minute essentials and did my best to pause the steady slideshow of possible frightening events, and my preplanned response to each one should they occur at some point during the fourteen hours that separated our bubble from the secure roots of home. No nostalgic pit stops were allowed, only required ones for fuel, Jazzy walks, and leg stretches as the doctor had ordered. Twilight softened the day and relief squeezed me tight when we finally slipped beneath the protective arms of our aging cottonwood guards.

Billy stepped out, stretched long and deep, sighed and locked his fingers into mine. Hand-in-hand we floated through the softness of August's evening warmth before we dropped onto the welcoming safety of the back steps. The thick scent of a Montana summer blended perfectly with the glowing hues of twilight and lit a flame of nerve-tingling memories. I squeezed up close and rested deep into his embrace, filling all sixty seconds of a full minute with the presence of him. Euphoria fell away with the rumblings of family, immediately drawing us into their world and filling our days with barbecues, fishing trips, and wedding plans. Kevin and Autumn had decided to exchange vows beneath the cottonwoods on the same family property where Billy and I had promised our hearts to one another years before, and the planning began instantly.

The monster was unable to penetrate the fortress of home for two full weeks. I whirled in a cloud of laughter and denial beneath the cottonwoods and an endless Montana sky with Billy at my side, and caught my breath when the last bag was stowed back into the trunk. The drive seemed long and Billy tired, resting into his music and watching the mountains and plains whiz past him. Fourteen hours were mostly silent. Only music. I prayed—another perfect fall, another holiday, a bit more time to frolic in the ordinary without a reminder from The Taker.

Billy's childlike apathy continued and grew once we settled back into our fragile bubble. He allowed me to shower and dress him, choose his meals, buckle his seatbelt and plan every activity with an oblivious air of contentment. He no longer made an attempt at household chores or created a walking stick to completion. The garage was filled with sticks he obsessively collected and I continued to encourage his attempt, though stripping the bark and stashing the naked little sticks in random corners was all he could manage. I held true to my vow. I never let him see my fear. We were on a wild adventure that would never end, and our perfect little world was just that—perfect. It was all he needed to know.

Though the duties of caregiving had become strenuous and progressive, I grew into them, intentionally grateful for the orchestra that continued to serenade me from beneath his chest. With each passing day I became more aware of The Giver's predestined melding of our souls from the moment we had met, and lost bits of time through years of selfish whims were now magnified by the fear of loss. My spirit cried out for a re-do, a rewind of time, a chance to replace the disdain he often met at the threshold of home with a grateful welcome to fill his deserving spirit with unconditional love. How often we forfeit the present day's joy, unaware of future longing and regret left floating in the wake of insignificant battles.

My dismal ponderings were squelched when Jack and Judi floated into our bubble with a Flathead Valley huckleberry pie and a bottle of wine, and Billy's giggle was infectious when she pulled another crisp Moose's Saloon cap out from behind her back and slipped it on top of his head.

Jack's interest in airplanes of any style led us the forty miles inland to McMinnville the next morning. It was hot outside and the air damp and heavy when we pulled into the lot of The Evergreen Aviation Museum, home to the original Spruce Goose. A symbol of American industry during World War II, the Spruce Goose is the largest plane ever constructed and made entirely of wood. Designed and built by Howard Hughes, it is also known as Hughes' Flying Boat. It flew only once, on November 2, 1947, at an altitude of seventy feet for only one minute. Many were doubtful that the giant wooden plane could actually fly, so it remained in a climate controlled hangar until the death of Howard Hughes in 1976. Finally in February of 1993, after a long barge ride up the Pacific Coast, and the Columbia and

Willamette Rivers, it found a home in the Evergreen Aviation Museum in McMinnville, Oregon, and Jack was eager to explore its interior.

Once inside the immense and spotless museum, Jack gave Billy a *follow me* wave and they disappeared amongst the vast display of war planes gleaming in restored grandeur. The huge vaulted ceiling met with a wall of glass that bounced daylight's brilliance off of the gleaming floor, illuminating the eerie dark history of war. Jack's enthusiasm only grew with the freshly purchased tickets for admittance into the monstrous Spruce Goose. Judi and I cautiously followed behind while Jack led Billy up the narrow steps to an opening that led into the plane's ghostly underbelly. Met by a tour guide waiting in the shadows, I slipped my hand into Billy's and was immediately drawn into fascinating details about the life of Howard Hughes and his most challenging endeavor. Billy and Jack were even allowed to sit briefly as make-believe pilot and co-pilot before we retraced our steps and followed one another down the narrow metal staircase and back onto the gleaming showroom floor.

The heavy heat spilling through the windows pushed us much more quickly through the remainder of the museum, and we finished with thirst-quenching wine samples from the Evergreen Vineyards. With a souvenir bottle of Pinot Gris boasting a Spruce Goose label tucked under our arms, we dropped into the air conditioned car and looked forward to a cool evening dinner at the beach.

Jack and Judi's journey would lead them north the next day, up Pacific Highway 101, and all the way into Washington where Jack's family would be waiting. But before we parted ways, Billy and I followed behind through the damp air of morning, thick with an earthy fragrance intensified by the sun's warmth, to Tillamook with plans for breakfast and a trip through the Tillamook Cheese Factory.

A self-guided tour found us bumping elbows with other curious tourists and dodging toddlers pushing their way through the crowd to smash themselves up against the wall of glass that allowed a view of the factory workers far below. Decked out in little plastic shower caps, aprons, and gloves, each employee manned a post that pushed blocks of fresh cheese through machines that trimmed, sliced and packaged them in captivating repetition. We finally pulled ourselves away from the glass and turned to another observatory of giant, nearly floor-to-ceiling, stainless steel capsules housing freshly made ice cream from the many local dairy farms belonging to the Tillamook dairy co-op.

Historical facts caught our attention on several plaques while shuffling our way through the large chaotic hall and back down the same shiny tiled staircase we had gone up. At the bottom, we immediately bumped into the back end of a compact line of tourists inching their way past an array of stainless steel tubs, each brimming with a variety of fresh cheese samples. A toothpick boasted one final, flavorful chunk of fresh cheese steadied between our fingers when the slow-moving line finally spit us out into a colorful gift shop overflowing with all things cow-or-cheese-related. We browsed a bit, giggled a lot, and quickly found the line that led us to a fresh Tillamook ice cream cone. Holding tight to a warm waffle cone wrapped in a napkin and dripping with cream, we bumped our way through the glass doors and directly into a rainy afternoon. Jack and Judi were now ready to face the rest of their drive north, so quick hugs in the misty rain etched another never-to-be-forgotten memory into my scrapbook.

The rainy afternoon was unable to dampen the optimistic air I took back to our bubble, and although the monster continued to incessantly nudge and taunt, I became more grateful with each passing day that the beautiful music of Billy's heart had not been interrupted for weeks, and waves of breath-catching anxiety had finally calmed some.

I started each morning intentional. I dodged the monster, kept my Billy close, hugged him often and observed him quietly. I created distractions, jotting down chores to finish up before the quiet fall gave way once again to the holidays and winter's gray. Tidy the garden beds, freshen the hot tub water, and make Billy an appointment with the eye doctor. He had made the request. He thought his eyes must be changing. I wanted so badly to see what he saw, or didn't see. Why did he guide his steps with an elbow against the wall? Why did he lean a bit? Why did he put his glasses up, then down, and then shift them around? What was that damn monster up to now? I made the appointment. November the thirteenth. Plenty of time to squeeze in my list of fall chores.

CHAPTER 21

MUSICAL INTERRUPTION

IN THE MIDST of routine, when our guard is down, spirit-altering events often explode the ordinary. September the nineteenth, 2013 became an *extra*ordinary day, vivid in my memory, and the search for simple words to describe a falling away of the physical to allow release of the spiritual is difficult.

I awoke alert, and fully aware of the day's surreal and dreamlike beginning. Fall's warmth led us into the peaceful harmony of the beach, toward Kyllo's, for an early birthday lunch on a sunlit patio. A slow, overwhelming awareness had drawn me into our surroundings. Pastel droplets of mist sparkled through translucent clouds and The Artist's already vibrant hues of silver, pink and blue glistened in supernatural brilliance. My fleshly shell seemed as light as the salt-laden air and a breath-catching shiver rose up from my depths and exited with an electric tingle that shook me when I grasped Billy's oblivious hand. I felt weightless, drenched in peace and vibrant color, and warmed with unconditional love. When the heaviness of my natural being eventually returned, my spirit was thirsty and far less content with the finite, and I was left to wonder if I had been allowed to wander tangibly near The Veil's edge. I carried remnants of uplifting peace across the day's boundaries and into the next twenty-four hours, unwittingly armed with the strength required to bear life's next revelation.

My birthday followed that extraordinary day and blurred them into a single forty-eight hour, unforgettable day. September the twentieth had an ordinary beginning, cluttered with ordinary moments until late in the afternoon when my phone rang. Danny was calling to see how Billy had handled the news. We hadn't heard. But then I had, and I was left with the burden of preventing or allowing life's sorrow. I turned to Billy and allowed him the right to life's sorrow. Woody's symphony had been silenced in sleep. Billy cried a brother's tears. Beth's spirit had been exploded into fragments she would gather together as remnants of her former self, and my extraordinary, forty-eight hour, spirit-altering birthday would forever be etched with the memory of Woody.

The silver lining of memory loss had lifted Billy's burden of sorrow by morning, but I struggled to emerge from my sadness and join him in *his* ordinary day. My heart ached for Beth and her son, and the awareness of my own impending heartache loomed larger while the monster sniffed and snarled around my Billy. I fought to keep our weakened bubble inflated, knowing my only defense was to love him absolutely, and not falter. My fall chore list dragged some of the ordinary back in and drew me deeper into Billy's presence again. I set my sadness aside and focused on staying one step ahead of the monster.

November the thirteenth crept up quickly and Billy was eager to have a brand new prescription for his glasses. A full exam required dilating drops and an exasperating array of questions to which Billy was unable to respond. His face drained pale with exhaustion when we finally pushed through the confines of the office and back out into the sunny parking lot. He shook his head, stretched his arms up high and yawned deeply before I buckled him in. I was assuring him of a warm lunch and a long nap when I pulled up to the stoplight at the highway's intersection. He was too quiet. I turned toward him to find his body slumped lifeless against his shoulder strap. Only *I* heard my panicked shriek,

"BILLY! No! No! No! Don't do this to me!"

I pulled off of the highway and reached over to free him from his seatbelt, when his arms once again flew out to the side and another bolt of electricity shocked the life back into his eyes. Exhaustion, confusion and panic had left us both weak and trembling. Another visit to the doctor left us with a referral to a cardiologist in Portland and the decision to implant a monitoring device early in December that would record his heartbeats for up to a year. Surgery, anesthesia, viruses, loss of consciousness are all detrimental to the demented brain, and another conquest for the monster. We were beginning to lose the war.

Stitched into a shallow pocket in his chest, just visible enough to remind me daily of its purpose, the device began capturing the music and any suspension of notes, the length of all fermatas in the composition at the discretion of The Conductor. I waited anxiously for signs of the next interruption.

Another Christmas season was soon plucked from my field of bountiful gifts. Levi popped through the revolving airport doors first, and, next, Autumn on the elbow of her fiancé. With a few reminders, Billy's recollection of which name belonged to which face jiggled into place and remained for bits of time. My name, Lisa Ann, had not yet been lost and was poetry to my ears whenever it wriggled its way through the tangles and past his lips.

Levi and Kevin had discovered an instant brotherly affection and their jovial banter was unexpected and entertaining. A slight release of motherly concern caught my attention when I witnessed Kevin's gentleness wrap itself around Autumn. Snuggled up there on the sofa, a steaming cup of cocoa in each of their hands, wrapped in the fluffy warmth of a winter's blanket and the reflection of twinkling Christmas lights, I knew. She would be safe with him. They would be kind to one another. My thoughts skipped ahead to a spring filled with the distraction of wedding preparations.

Droplets of gratefulness blended with the crystal air of Christmas in our failing bubble and I breathed in the healthy burst deeply before the continual momentum of time sucked it all back through those revolving airport doors. Levi was the last to go, and an extra tight, apprehensive hug preceded the usual wink and kiss before he disappeared. A year's time had brought obvious and ominous change, and distance had left Levi and Autumn feeling helpless.

The holiday washed a pale fatigue over Billy's face and I looked forward to our usual stop in Sherwood for a strong cup of coffee before we finished our trip home from the airport. He sat quietly, yawning and pale, sipping slowly from his steaming cup. I studied him. His head bobbed some. We were halfway between the cardiologist and our bubble, and a quick call to the device clinic had us turned around and waiting for a monitoring report within the hour.

The printer clicked off page after page. Billy sat wired to the machine while I watched the monitor display his rhythm. And then it didn't. Nothing. A thin green line, but Billy sat upright and awake. I wondered if the machine had faltered or if the symphony had paused. I went for the nurse, but the doctor came instead. He had just interpreted the first pages of the clicking report and explained in an astonished tone that Billy's heart had paused for over ten seconds - *several times*. A pacemaker was implanted that evening. The pesky arrhythmia had been caught and remedied. His natural pacemaker had been misfiring and the mechanical one would now step in when needed. The orchestra should play uninterrupted. The new year would begin.

CHAPTER 22

BITTERSWEET

JAMIE AND MOLLY'S home had been our refuge through surgery and follow-up appointments, and Billy's body healed quickly. The symphony's steady melody left his cheeks a rosy red. He sparkled more, but spoke less. One victory had not reclaimed ground from battles lost. He clung to me and grew fearful if I wasn't near. Television bewildered him, crowds confused him, and family chaos most often annoyed him.

We hadn't been out in a while and because Billy's love for car rides and shopping had become adorable and childlike, we left Jazzy with Molly and went out into the world for an afternoon of browsing and fresh air. Warding off panic's onset should I blend too deeply into the sea of shoppers, I hovered nearby like an overprotective parent, allowing him to wander between aisles, bouncing from one distraction to another. Every store had become a treasure trove of trinkets and he had stored up a fine collection of shiny wrist watches, and a variety of brightly colored miniature flashlights and tiny metallic pocket knives. I caught myself smiling, submerged in a parent-like love, giddy with gratefulness for the freshly borrowed time The Giver had recently lent, when suddenly guilt squeezed through and illuminated my selfish joy. The orchestra's mechanical assistant had spared me the pain of sudden loss, but the bittersweet trade had lengthened

Billy's war and given the monster indefinite access to his remaining bits. My thoughts were wandering through a forest of *what-ifs* and *should-or-shouldn't-haves*, when my phone rang again.

Molly wanted us home.

"Jazzy just tipped over," were her exact words. "She doesn't look good."

Again? Really? Within the hour we were waiting in the vet clinic. Three hundred dollars and an electrolyte injection later, she rested on Molly's kitchen floor while we watched and waited for another miraculous recovery that wasn't happening. Her breathing was slow and heavy, she was shivering. I waited a bit longer. She grew colder, more still. I gathered her into a warm blanket and Molly and I rushed her to the nearby vet hospital through the dark January rain. A code of some kind was yelled through the office at the sight of her and she was whisked away to the emergency room. We waited. We had left Billy under the watchful eye of Jamie, and two hours had passed when the doctor finally summoned us into a private consultation room.

"This doesn't sound good," I whispered to Molly.

The doctor's voice was calm and she made it clear that Jazzy was in the midst of a serious crisis. If we had waited five minutes more we would have lost her. Her liver enzymes were through the roof. A possible allergic reaction, perhaps liver failure, or an unidentified liver disease could have been the cause. She would need to remain in intensive care for a few days.

I loved Jazzy, but my rational ears were drowning out the doctor's explanation with the sound of, *ChaChing! ChaChing! ChaChing!* The dollar signs bouncing around in my mind were replaced with a picture of Jazzy running pug shuffles through the sand or tugging at the end of her leash, and I reluctantly signed the consent form. She and Billy were inseparable, and once again my broken give-a-shit allowed me to throw financial concerns out the window. Save Jazzy! For Billy! What else could I do?

Three days and two thousand dollars later, Jazzy was free and bouncing with good health. We would need to have her liver evaluated when her enzymes were at normal levels, and she may need a monthly shot that would no doubt cost around one hundred and fifty dollars with each injection, was the doctor's assumption.

"Um, Not happening!" was my silent response to that assumption, "If she tips over again, its lights out for Jazzy!"

I watched her diet, gave her plenty of water and snuggles, and hoped for the best. Billy barely comprehended the entire ordeal and I alone prepared myself for the loss of Jazzy should she actually have an unidentified and possibly fatal liver issue. My mind was set and we continued in the bliss of the ordinary.

I looked around the interior of our precious bubble when we returned. We had been away long enough for it to have gained that forlorn, ghostly feel. I warmed it up, switched on some lights and turned open the blinds to the dusk of late afternoon. It was dreary. Our once brilliant, effervescent bubble was dreary, and in an instant I knew it was time to go. A stirring—one we all get at times if we are brave enough to acknowledge it—was churning in the pit of me. The illusion of co-existing for many years alongside a sluggish monster had been shattered. Our monster was not sluggish. He was ravenous and ill-tempered, always threatening to claim the spoils of war, which I had decided would happen on the battlefield of home. The monster roared a haughty echo off of the butter-colored walls while I planned our escape.

My new strategy brought with it a bright yellow "Property for Sale" sign that blocked the royal purple blossoms of Billy's young butterfly bush, and greeted us snidely each time we pulled into the driveway. I planned our escape for April, giving the shackles of winter time to fall away. Bursts of happy confetti drifted through the air with wedding details and kept our bubble afloat while we waited. I stitched together brightly colored bunting, shopped for a pretty mother-of-the-bride dress, and bought giant pastel daisies to adorn a wedding arch my nieces were designing. I laughed with my Billy, shared coffee and foggy mornings with him beneath the shelter of the porch, watched the roaring winter surf from the comfort of the car, and fell asleep to the music playing softly beneath the rise and fall of his warm chest. I mocked and shunned the monster while we waited, always fiercely aware of the last times dropping away like wilted flower petals.

It was soon time to put all of the *things* we had gathered through a shared life together back into boxes in preparation for the next season. Each room, the office, the kitchen cabinets, and the garage suddenly seemed swollen with life's baggage and I began to mentally assess each item for function or fluff. I no longer desired the bulkiness of fluff and began its eradication, and with the exception of a few sentimental items, the local second-hand store became the recipient of all things fluff-related. It left me feeling much lighter and, knowing it made little sense, also a bit more prepared for our final battle.

We stuffed the little orange Grand Prix from floorboards to sun roof again, leaving just enough room for Jazzy to squeeze between Billy and me. So, with fingers crossed for a quick sale and much work lying ahead in Montana, we left the rest of our worldly possessions temporarily behind and drove straight into our last season together. Billy's symphony continued, and I had been able to gently add each new *wait and see* symptom into the medley of other symptoms awaiting identification and remedy, allowing me to face that final season with forced hope and renewed strength in the sanctuary of home.

CHAPTER 23

THE BEST DAY EVER!

THE MONTH OF May in Montana was riddled with new patient consultations and symptom investigations, and although we were graciously welcomed into the country house with Papa and Donna, it took weeks of laborious efforts between Billy's appointments to minimize, rearrange, and mingle function and fluff into comfortable cohabitation. A new cardiologist and a new internist were becoming acquainted with the trickiness and stealth of Billy's monster. His blood pressure would spike and fall at random intervals, and although the orchestra continued to play uninterrupted, it struggled with a sporadically rapid tempo. But we settled in, and planned to retrieve the remainder of our world after Kevin and Autumn's *Best Day Ever,* which was scheduled for the twenty-eighth afternoon in June.

The transformation from spring to summer had spread a carpet of green velvet beneath our feet and an umbrella of apple blossoms and fragrant lilacs above our heads. Billy bounced around my heels, dodging sprinklers and romping with Jazzy while the bustle of wedding preparations swirled all around us. He now lived fully in each moment, unaware of the most recent moment that had fallen away and unconcerned with what the next one may bring. Oblivion and apathy were his consistent companions and I began to also find the grace in that. He seemed joyful, blissfully unaware. I watched him play in the delicious freshness of summer, dripping in green and brightened by the blue of a brilliant Montana sky. But the monster continued to nip at my Billy, leaving me in frequent silent prayer that by four o'clock, on the twenty-eighth afternoon of June, with Autumn locked at the elbows between them, her brother and her daddy would be able to walk her down an aisle of emerald green to an altar beneath the cottonwoods.

There are no words to explain the cauldron of artistic energy bubbling between my nieces, and I simply needed to nod my approval to each endearing prop and detail they meticulously designed, painted, and requested for addition into Autumn's big day. I gave their creativity full rein and jumped into the dirty work with Clint and Lisa. We trimmed trees, mowed lawns, added flower pots of color, and finished the weekends covered in dust with a cold beer in our hands. It was fun--tiring, fun, dirty work, and Billy laughed, a lot.

Autumn arrived with the winding down of details. Just a few remained and my spirit began feasting on the sight of my tiny bride-to-be floating by in her sundress and flip-flops, planting kisses on the cheek of her childlike father, and joining her cousins in the frenzy of last minute preparations for her wedding day. Tents were propped up and tables were adorned with burlap runners and mason jars of freshly cut daisies. Eye-catching photos were displayed amongst pyramids of fresh strawberry jam and honey sparkling atop hay bales stacked near the reception's entrance. Our decorating fairies had twinkle lights wrapped around the limbs of tall trees and swinging in the breeze above a checkerboard dance floor. One hundred sparkling white chairs waited in a sea of green to welcome those precious to us, and a winding aisle of flower petals led to the wedding arch, dressed and waiting beneath bowing cottonwoods. The entire yard was draped in *fancy country,* brimming with laughter and buckets of smiling daisies.

The big day arrived with an anxious reminder of the weather's power over an outdoor wedding. Swirling dust-devils spun rudely amongst guests kicking up bridesmaids' dresses and tablecloths, and tousling a few freshly lacquered hair-dos. And one of June's notorious thunderstorms began to brew on the eastern horizon, so we battened down the hatches of the tents in preemptive preparation.

Billy was perky and cooperative when I slipped him into his crisp new suit and tied his spring-colored tie. But, every now and then he gave me a puzzled look that signaled a needed reminder of the occasion, and with a final wink and an "Oh, yeah," he moseyed outside to be caught up into a welcoming cloud of not-seen-often-enough family. He bounced between his brothers, mothers, sisters, aunts and cousins. Fresh *new* leaves of our growing family tree continued to arrive and blended in effortlessly while the chaotic melody of family chatter rang through the air.

At precisely four o'clock in the afternoon, The Giver ordered the threatening thunderclouds and obnoxious dust-devils to be still, and a golden dome of sunshine brightened the baby blue of bridesmaids' dresses and the crisp yellow ties of groomsmen as they began their slow march past adoring faces, smiling from the rows of the stark white chairs. Soft notes of love songs floated beneath the cottonwood guardians, and tears slipped down my cheeks when Levi took one of his sister's elbows into his and gently adjusted his father's into her other. They stood regally at the top of the concrete staircase overlooking the winding aisle of flower petals and rows of patiently waiting family and friends. Autumn's tiny gown of delicate lace swooshed through the petals around her feet, allowing just the tips of her bright blue wedding shoes to peek through. Her wispy veil mingled with golden ringlets in a gentle June breeze and a proud smile lit up her sparkling blue eyes. Her daddy was walking her down the aisle. She silently acknowledged his physical presence and an aura of joy carried her into Kevin's welcoming arms.

Moments later my daughter had become a wife, and the instant peace I found in her new beginning tempered the pangs of my nearby ending. My spirit felt like dancing, and I did. The afternoon glow melted into soft twilight and with twinkle lights swaying in the breeze and lighting up the dance floor, I watched from the comfort of Levi's embrace when Autumn took the hand of her father and let him lead her in out-of-step rhythm to the music. Joy and pain had become inseparable roommates in my heart.

Molly's effervescence quickly drew a crowd of participation onto the dance floor and we bounced and reveled for hours beneath glowing tents and evening shadows. It truly was *The Best Day Ever.*

CHAPTER **24**

THE BEGINNING OF THE END

AN UNOFFICIAL PEACE treaty with the monster ended with June. Billy's new doctor was now on an intense mission to understand the cause of his random and dangerously high blood pressure and heart rate spikes. Bloodwork and stress tests ordered by the cardiologist eliminated any involvement of the orchestra and other chambers of his body were soon under scrutiny. An endocrinologist was consulted and his thyroid examined. More bloodwork and ultrasounds tossed that theory into the medley of wait and see symptoms, and that is what we continued to do, wait and see.

While we waited and continually monitored and recorded blood pressure readings, we squeezed in a fishing trip to Tiber Reservoir with Clint and Lisa. Wedding plans had not allowed time for fishing trips in June and we were eager to take Billy out in hopes of helping him catch a walleye or two, and relieve the stresses of continual poking and prodding.

The July weekend started out hot and grew hotter. We pitched the tent, stowed the coolers and climbed aboard the boat in anticipation of a cool afternoon boat ride and an abundance of fish. Billy was excited and held his precious Moose's Saloon cap on tightly through the cool and windy boat ride to one of Clint's favorite fishing coves. He was no longer able to rig his own pole or maintain the patience or focus necessary to keep the line in the water, so I became his fishing partner. We shared in the chore of slipping worm after worm onto the hook as well as the joy of reeling in a few walleye for hours under the hot July sun.

As the heat grew more intense, Billy became antsy. I dipped his cap into the cool water of the lake and slipped it back onto his head in hopes of keeping his body temperature stable. He shook his head and shoulders and squealed at the frigid water dripping down his overheated cheeks. Expecting him to giggle and relax in relief, I was surprised when he became anxious and consumed with fear instead. In an instant he had no idea where he was or who *we* were. He was scared to death, flailing his arms and begging for us to take him home. We stowed the poles, Clint fired up the engine and we turned the boat toward camp. He tried to reel Billy in with humor, chuckled and said,

"Hey Big Fella, ya wanna sit on my lap and steer?"

Billy's exasperated response was a breathless,

"Nooooo thank you!" and he began to slam his fists on the side of the boat.

His behavior became even more erratic and unmanageable; forcing us to stop at the marina, halfway between Clint's fishing cove and camp. With the hope of dry ground snapping Billy out of his frightening hallucination, we coaxed him out of the boat and onto the dock. He ranted and pulled away several times before we were able to guide him up the steep and rocky hill leading to the shelter of the marina. He was convinced that the marina was a loony bin and we were dropping him off there, so he spun around and darted out the door just as soon as we stepped through it. Passersby outside were then hailed with rude and unsavory remarks, leaving me to calm the ire of a few beer and ego-driven country boys. My heart was pounding. We were in the middle of nowhere. I was ill-equipped and unprepared, and panic held me in a tight grip.

Clint and Lisa left me squeezing Billy's hand at a picnic table in the shade while they sped back to camp in the boat intending to retrieve us with the car. I waited, gently urging Billy to calm down, tugging him back to the picnic table whenever he jerked away in an attempt to escape. I kept my voice calm, tried to maintain contact with his darting and fear-filled eyes. I wanted to hold him and tell him everything was alright but he was afraid of me, convinced that I intended him harm. My heart was breaking and panic left me weak. Where was Clint? It was only a few miles. Billy's head jerked toward the bright orange Grand Prix when Clint finally pulled up in a cloud of dust. He darted a doubtful look at me when I tried to convince him that Clint was there to take us home. His eyes held no trust, but the word *home* allowed me to slowly guide him into the backseat. We locked the doors and turned the air conditioner up as high as it would go. Was it the heat? Was it the cold water I had irresponsibly doused his head with?

"Is Mom there?" he asked. "How about Dad, will he be there? And Grandma Florence?"

His eyes continued to dart around. He picked up a magazine and commented on a conspiracy peering back at him from its cover before he angrily tossed it to the floorboards. The few miles over the dusty gravel road back to camp seemed to stretch out forever. We finally pulled up next to our campsite and scrambled out of the car in preparation of Billy's next outburst, but his stunned expression when he saw his favorite camp chair and the fire pit instantly shocked him back into our world. His face relaxed, his tense muscles drooped and he turned to me.

"How did you do that?" he asked. "It's like magic!"

I was baffled. He was back, spoke so clearly, and had no recollection of the hellish hour we had just endured. I held him before we sank into the comfort of the camp chairs to gather our bearings. A restless night in the tent was followed by an eager and early departure back to civilization. Overnight fishing trips were forever banned. One more painful last time had fallen away.

The doctor's bitter explanation of the experience was difficult to digest. An anti-psychotic medication would be kept on hand and administered should Billy need to be medically reined in when the monster temporarily possessed his reality again. Not *if*, but *when*. It was the beginning of the end, with no end in sight. I would love him, protect him, and fearfully wait.

CHAPTER **25**

COCOONING

INSTINCTS ARE POWERFUL, maternal instincts supernaturally so. The Giver had stirred my joyful spirit into nesting before the births of Levi and Autumn, but this time the churning in the pit of me was dark and urgent, sparked by The Taker, and I began spinning a secure cocoon where Billy and I could wait out our last season.

Movers were scheduled to meet us at our bubble the third week of July. I rallied my reliable troops, and with Clint and Billy in the cockpit of a giant rented suburban, and Lisa, Savana, and I tucked in next to two jittery toddlers behind them, we set out with plans to transfer the remainder of our bubble into my freshly spun cocoon. We were on guard throughout the fourteen hour drive, prepared for battle but praying for peace. I strategically placed myself within arm's reach directly behind Billy and reached around the headrest often to stroke his cheek or squeeze his shoulder in anxious hope that the consistent reminder of my presence would keep him grounded and the monster at bay. It seemed to work. The monster napped.

My heart jumped at the sight of our lonely little house, and fell just as quickly when that smug "Property for Sale" sign, still blocking the view of Billy's butterfly bush, caught my eye. Once inside, Molly and the girls instantly strengthened my troops with laughter, and surprising bursts of my Billy began to pop out and entertain us.

He played and laughed, wore funny hats and jumped on the beds with Savana's wee ones. Once the loading of worldly possessions was complete, we finished the moving day with a giggle-filled slumber party on air mattresses in the living room of our deflated bubble.

Billy seemed happy to be *home*. Guilt dropped by again. Had I confused him with our retreat to Montana? Had my fearful escape left him with a longing to go home? Was our bubble now the last home he recalled and yearned for? I tried to reassure myself that he had very little awareness of his surroundings from day to day, but at the same time wondered if that were true. More guilt piled up with the fear that perhaps it wasn't. What was he feeling? I was always left to wonder.

The moving truck weighted down with our world, rumbled around the corner the following morning and we filled the remaining hours of the day at the beach. Clint and Lisa built sandcastles and danced in the waves with their grandchildren while Molly and Savana captured every delicious moment with their cameras.

Billy and I were watching from the cozy comfort of our sun-warmed blanket when he reached out and cupped my face between his hands. He stared into my eyes, pure joy lighting up his entire face. He tried to speak, but stuttered. He shook his head and tried again. His soft words fell slowly.

"Will you marry me?" he asked.

He loved me, and was hoping to begin a brand new life with me, completely unaware that we were nearing the end of a full life we had already shared. Pain and joy collided head on again.

"We are already married, Billy," I replied.

His expression was priceless.

"WOW! Really?" was his disbelieving response.

"Yes, my Billy. For nearly twenty-eight years now," I explained.

He pulled me close, kissed me long and held me tight. The dark bitter sweetness settled deep. The salty air had made him sleepy and he stretched out on the blanket, a contented sigh escaped and he closed his eyes. I watched him and could not contain my sorrow. My tears mixed with the salt and sand. Molly sat down next to me and wrapped an arm around my shoulders. Another last time was wilting and nearly ready to fall away. Billy and I would never share another playful afternoon on the Oregon Coast. Our memories would end there. I knew that. He didn't. Molly and I watched the rolling waves in silence.

I snubbed the sneering bright yellow "Property for Sale" sign when we pulled away from our precious bubble. My breath fought hard to get through the tightness in my throat and I squeezed Billy's hand when we turned onto Highway 101 and slipped into the tunnel of towering Oregon pines that had once welcomed us into our new world. It had been surreal and finite. Anger hammered away the tears and I refused to look back.

It was well into the night when our caravan crept through the shadows beneath the familiar cottonwood canopy, and we were weary. Our final season would begin with the arrival of dawn.

CHAPTER 26

A FINAL SEASON

OUR WORLDLY TREASURES arrived shortly after we did and were temporarily stuffed into the safety of a storage unit, and with the help of Lisa and her generous children they were filtered, condensed, and squeezed into our cocoon before August's end.

Because fall and winter often sneak into Montana hand-in-hand and can be rather mischievous, and visions of drifting snow had become tangled up with dark forebodings churning in my pit, I began a mission to stuff our cocoon with a stockpile of snowbound essentials. The darkness lifted some with Billy's thrill of pitching unusual items randomly into the shopping cart in toddler-like fashion. Sometimes he shot me a questioning look for approval; other times he tossed a simple desire into the heap defiantly, with an unspoken dare to stop him. It was comical, and I continued to indulge his every whim.

"You can have whatever you want, Billy," was my standard response, which he often confirmed with a confident nod.

Society's rules and boundaries no longer applied to my Billy and pocket checks were required before leaving each store. A miffed pout followed when I retrieved gum, mints, candy bars or trinkets from jacket and jean pockets and returned to the checkout to keep us both honest. He whistled through the parking lot. He still whistled. That fascinated me.

The little Grand Prix was once again stuffed floorboards to sunroof with comforts intended to ease the angst of winter. With our cocoon prepared for our final season, we went outside to play in the warmth of summer's last days.

Until the monster awoke from his nap. He was groggy at first and only snarled through Billy in spurts. He would make Billy curse, threaten, and throw things; and I would follow nearby, waiting patiently for a temporary retreat.

Between the nasty spurts, we stacked firewood, picked apples, and raked up mountains of dusty golden leaves throughout the colorful crispness of fall. But a frigid Montana winter soon blew in and the monster grew angrier. I was able to tame it with medication at first, but before long Billy had become a prisoner of war and I was allowed only rare visits. I struggled to shed the heavy weights of fear and fatigue, and with each increased dose of antipsychotics I grew more aware that we were nearing the end of this dark war.

Thanksgiving brought Kevin and Autumn through deep snow and dangerous wind chills for a final holiday with Billy, and Levi brightened up our cocoon when he flew in on Christmas Day. But the holiday season held no glitter for me. There were no gifts left waiting in green fields ahead.

The new year began more fearfully than the previous one had ended. Papa was hospitalized with kidney failure around the same time I began searching for a safe haven for my Billy. Papa's kidneys rebounded just before a discovery of bladder cancer spun him into a whirlwind of surgery and chemotherapy, and the bright yellow "Property for Sale" sign had finally beckoned a buyer for our bubble, so in early February our season at the beach officially ended. More bitter sweet.

The forest in Billy's brain had become dark and twisted, a shelter befitting his monster's demeanor and he paced—angry, restless and frightened. The monster would bind my Billy amongst the tangles for hours at a time, leaving me to wait patiently for a glimmer of his true spirit to reappear through his soft blue eyes. I embraced those bits of time and used them wisely, but soon realized that my desire to care for Billy on my own had become unrealistic, perhaps even selfish. If only love and courage were enough.

The thought of releasing Billy's daily care into an army of professionals overwhelmed me and I called Jamie. I needed a trusted comrade. He eased my burden and arrived in early March to spend a final weekend with his brother and help me seek a safe haven. We were both naïve and unaware at the time that such a place did not exist.

Jamie waited with Billy while I prepared myself for a morning tour. Once we had left Billy under the watchful eye of nervous family members and our journey was underway, Jamie's intrigue spilled over. He explained the curious behavior he had witnessed as he waited in silence with his brother. Billy was usually oblivious, barely able to speak, often fearful and in his own world. But when his favorite music began to play, he chimed in. Jamie sat in quiet awe when Billy began to sing along, clearly reciting the lyrics to *Harvest Moon*, one of his all-time favorites. Those moments spent alone with his brother had left behind the gift of a peaceful and final memory he would carry back to Oregon with him.

The safe haven Jamie and I finally agreed upon was wrapped up beautifully in cozy comforts of an artificial home. Soft lighting enhanced a stylish dining room that guaranteed healthy home-cooked meals, and snazzy paintings adorned a perimeter of *safety* within which confused residents could safely roam. French doors opened into a sunlit atrium that sat proudly in the center, allowing freedom to the outdoors without the threat of danger, and the studio apartment they would prepare for my Billy was spotless and well-decorated. A large sunny window looked out to the atrium and we were encouraged to add personal photos and treasures to the already tasteful décor. We were assured that the caregivers were compassionate and fully trained in the areas of dementia and geriatrics, and they greeted us sweetly as we toured the halls. From the outside looking in they appeared compassionate and capable of managing the monster's outbursts as we had been assured they were.

It sounded too good to be true, and we sat in emotional turmoil across from Mr. Marketing Director, wanting desperately to muster faith in his convincing speech. He pointed out that there was a waiting list for the highly coveted room situated securely behind the locked doors of the memory care unit, and we shouldn't wait too long as the monster was unpredictable and the room was being held especially for my Billy. Noting I was not yet convinced, he continued to explain that with proper direction there was a possibility that angry outbursts may not only be managed, but eliminated; and the staff included registered nurses, experienced in the areas of dementia and geriatrics and available twenty-four hours every day to assist and guide the caregivers.

Mr. Marketing Director allowed us time alone. I turned my tear-stained face to Jamie for guidance. We shared the same fears. Billy was no longer safe at home with his monster, yet releasing the reins as caregiver left me spinning with guilt and doubt. We hesitantly agreed to Billy's new home. As we drove away, Jamie joked that Mr. Marketing Director could probably sell ice cubes to an Eskimo. He had, and our decision will haunt me for the remainder of my life.

CHAPTER **27**

GUARDS FOR THE MONSTER

MARCH THE SIXTEENTH, the first day of the last days. Lisa and I took Billy to lunch. He loved cheeseburgers and he was happy to be out. The sun was shining and his new room was waiting, dressed up with family photos and his favorite treasure boxes. His Moose's Saloon cap hung from a hook on the closet door and his favorite Oregon Ducks blanket was draped over the love seat. It should have felt a bit like home, but from the moment we stepped through the door he seemed to know. He dropped his head and I watched the panic wash over him. What had I done? But what could I do? The caregiver assigned to my Billy for the first twenty-four hours attempted to draw him into his new environment with a soft slow tone, but he knew. I was abandoning him and he knew. I panicked, my spirit was screaming. I stepped toward him, ready to grab his hand and run, but That Nurse motioned for me to follow her into the hallway. My memory's lens captured Billy's expression of fear and betrayal as I turned away and it burned permanently into my mind's eye. I left Billy with the caregiver and followed That Nurse to a comfortable chair in the hall. She immediately began a failed attempt at reassurance that he would be well-protected and that *separation* would be good for both of us. The transition needed to begin right then. She was not fully aware of the addictive love we had for one another and the withdrawal that would follow. But Billy needed a fortress for his monster, with experienced guards at the door, and I left him behind the walls of promised protection. The tearing away twisted me inside and unexpected grief poured out. I leaned into Lisa's comforting embrace as she led me through the parking lot. The doubt and guilt began their consumption of me and I felt nauseous. I feared that I had left Billy in a cage with his monster and I fought hard against the urge to run back in and save him.

Within hours my addiction forced me to check in, praying that he didn't miss me. I didn't want him to miss me. I was prepared for him to prefer his new home to *our* home, and with the assurance that Billy was settled quietly for the night, I snuggled deep into the softness of a blanket and succumbed to heartbreak.

The first week without him next to me brought with it a physical pain that I had not been prepared for, and every day and every night for one full week progress reports were given. The monster had been contained and Billy was wandering safely through the halls of his new home. Photos sent frequently were proof that he was eating, and smiling, and perhaps adjusting. He had even danced once to music playing in the sunlit sitting room. Mr. Marketing Director insisted that I could rest, and I tried.

Friday, I was going to see my Billy on Friday. Five days without me would be enough, and I called to make lunch plans for Friday. My plans were dashed. That Nurse suggested that Billy meet the weekend staff before I interrupted the progress of the very sensitive transition. I would trust That Nurse for two more days—after all, photos were continually reassuring. My Billy was safe. I would wait.

Monday, March the twenty third, I had never been so excited to see my Billy. Autumn and Kevin had come for the first visit, and Autumn was eager to see her daddy and his new home. An early birthday lunch would be a perfect celebration. But more heartbreak was waiting behind the locked door to the memory care unit. Autumn, Kevin, and I found Billy slumped in an armchair in that same sunlit

145

sitting room, his eyes closed, drool pooling onto the soft red polo shirt Grandma Joyce had given him for Christmas. He wasn't wearing his glasses. I asked where they were. A caregiver found them in the kitchen—twisted, broken and dirty. Autumn snatched them and went in search of a repair shop. I went in search of answers.

Billy had not slept well was the answer I received. Anxiety medication was required which left him lethargic and drooling most of that unfortunate Monday. My Billy had retreated back into the tangles and he was unaware that I had returned. He would not recognize his baby girl or share a birthday lunch with her. Questions were bouncing around in my guilt-ridden brain. Had they lied to me for an entire week? Was the monster already unmanageable? Why hadn't they called me over the weekend? The fragment of confidence I was frantically holding onto fell to the bottom of my fear pit and I once again fought the urge to grab his hand and run. But where would I go? We weren't safe anywhere; and that damn monster was everywhere.

The following two days were the *last* two days I had any hope at all of regaining the tiniest bit of confidence in the professional ability of those I had chosen to care for my Billy. I attempted to convince myself that the *transition* could take time, but hope and trust evaporated quickly.

I watched him sleeping. The monster's roar had once again required sedation during the nighttime hours and had left Billy droopy and napping through most of the day. It was the twenty-sixth of March, his fifty-eighth birthday. I had high hopes for laughter and treasured moments of clarity, but it was not to be. The day was nearly done, as was the second week of the gut-wrenching *transition*.

I took in his radio. The caregivers there had discovered his love for nearly every genre of music. Perhaps it would quiet the monster. That one time he had danced, and they had giggled. That one time I had hope. When sedation wore off I held him long, and he was calm. I calmed him. How is it possible to love another human being so deeply? I attempted to replace lost bits of myself every day as I drank in his physical presence and absorbed his spirit through each long embrace. I slipped my arms under his, wrapped them tightly around him and whispered softly into his ear, "I will love you forever, Billy. Remember." His full weight relaxed against my chest.

Week three brought no relief. Billy's monster didn't play well with others, and many of his demented neighbors were incapable of rational responses to the monster's taunts. So, because physical or verbal confrontations often occurred in the evening while the caregivers were busy clearing dinner dishes, mopping floors and doing the laundry, I began staying after dinner and late into the evening, preempting battles and sedation. Carpet lined the perimeter my Billy endlessly wandered, and I wondered if his medicated eyes were adjusting to the dizzying pattern with which oblivious decorators had smattered his surroundings. I pondered while pacing on his elbow one evening, and I paused to clear the fruit cocktail filling the lenses of reading glasses dangling from a chain around the neck of a frail little wheelchair-bound woman. She had been waiting patiently to be readied for bed. Why were the caregivers doing dishes and mopping floors while this tiny, frail little woman waited for a kind hand to remove the fruit cocktail from her glasses? I wondered why the thousands of dollars per month, per resident, of this facility dripping with ambiance was not enough to cover the costs of regularly scheduled kitchen help. Were other family members concerned or had they not spent enough time there to notice? Is dignity not awarded to the elderly or mentally impaired? I had never found myself in the bowels of a care facility before and awareness slapped me hard across the cheek. A fancy package had camouflaged the common practice of neglect when the constant presence of an advocate is absent, and compassion sold at the gate was lost in the interior. The dishes needed to be stacked. The floors needed to be mopped. The towels needed laundering. The frail little woman would wait, with lenses filled with fruit cocktail.

Failed promises from trained professionals in the fields of geriatrics and dementia soon forced me into the position of full-time caregiver once again, in the very environment intended to relieve my constant vigilance over Billy's safety and quality of life. The monster's nastiness continued to leave the caregivers unwilling to engage in battle over personal hygiene duties. But Billy allowed me to shower, shave, and dress him, and I greedily accepted the challenge. I loved being near him, and sometimes if I held his face in my hands and looked deep into his eyes, he seemed to see me. Sometimes he hugged me back. Sometimes he smiled. Sometimes he said thank you. He could still peek out from behind the tangles—sometimes.

By the end of week three the transition had still shown no promise, and I was a millisecond away from *breaking him out* with a renewed determination to face each battle on my own. My strength, and love for this man, had been grossly underestimated by those with one foot in the trenches and the other clinging to their rung of the corporate ladder. They had taken notice of my constant presence. I had become a mole in their understaffed operation and a guard to the monster's guards.

CHAPTER **28**

A DOWNHILL SLIDE

SITTING WITH HIM through dinner one Thursday evening at the start of April, he barely ate and winced in pain with every swallow. They hadn't noticed his discomfort nor offered a remedy. *I* made the request for pain relief. His discomfort had allowed only a short nap earlier that afternoon, leaving the monster to roar and pace unattended when he awoke and I had not yet returned to stand guard. He had squeezed the finger of a caregiver and threatened to break the forearm of another staff member during my short absence. Billy was young and still strong, and the fragile caregivers were no match for his monster. What if I had taken the restful vacation that had been confidently suggested at the onset of the transition? Would he have prowled in pain through the night as well? The Tylenol helped some. He slept soon after dinner. I would cautiously wait.

Friday, April the third, a sunny spring morning lit up the dining room. I coaxed Billy into eating a tiny bit of breakfast. He wasn't feeling well and was eager for his morning nap. Lunchtime found him the same, sleepy and uncomfortable. I requested more Tylenol. They again obliged, at *my* request. They appeared unconcerned with his obvious discomfort. They now counted on my presence and shunned their scheduled duties further. Leaving him to nap in the afternoon warmth pouring through his window, I drove around aimlessly, afraid to stray too far.

I found myself winding through the shadows of the local cemetery searching for the headstone of Beth's baby boy, laid to rest there so many years before. I sat cross-legged on the damp grass in front of the stone bearing his name, unsure of what drew me there. I closed my eyes and absorbed the stillness. I prayed for Beth and for my Billy. I prayed for myself, and allowed my tears. A gentle breeze rustled a few lone leaves that had clung on tightly through the winter. They were strong. I needed to be strong. I ran my hands over the cool marble. My fingers traced the letters of his name, and I silently hoped that Beth wouldn't mind my intrusion into her private pain. I traced the date of his birth, April the third. I had been drawn to his resting place on the very date of his birth. It was Friday, April the third, baby Trenton's birthday. A day of prayer, and that peaceful breeze stirred me.

The spell was broken with the ringing of my phone. That Nurse had called to discuss Billy's medication adjustments due to the monster's angry outbursts the previous afternoon. It was nearly 4:00 in the afternoon when I arrived to meet That Nurse and found Billy stumbling around on his own, his head drooping, drooling, and barely able to swallow. He had been highly sedated to prevent further outbursts and was stepping high over thresholds and those dizzying patterns in the carpet. What must he have been seeing? How lost must he have felt? More guilt.

That Nurse finally informed me late into that Friday afternoon that she had spoken with Billy's psychiatrist the day before and a mood stabilizer had been added to his regimen without my knowledge. They had already administered two doses along with the antipsychotics and anxiety medication they had been doling out like Skittles, and yet it was *I* who needed to make the request for simple pain relief. I reluctantly left Billy in their oblivious hands long enough to pick up lozenges for his painful throat. But before I left, I checked a list of side effects for the newly prescribed medication, only to discover that a severe sore throat was a side effect that warranted a call to the doctor.

Had That Nurse not noticed his sore throat? Had That Nurse checked for side effects? That Nurse hadn't allowed *me* the opportunity to guard his reaction to a new drug. That Nurse had now lost all credibility. That Nurse had chosen late Friday afternoon to include me in Billy's care and the doctor's office was closed for the weekend by the time I was able to call for guidance. That Nurse would leave promptly for the weekend too, and I ran back into the monster's cage before she had a chance to grab her keys and escape. I found her in the hallway and insisted a hold be put on the new medication until the doctor could be consulted on Monday. She agreed to my request and instructed the med-tech to put a hold order into the computer system. Anger and relief joined me at the dinner table with Billy, where I needed to ask more than once for Tylenol for his discomfort. They finally returned with a spoonful of yogurt filled with crushed Tylenol. That was all he would swallow for dinner. I felt helpless amongst those who promised to be helpful.

Swallowing had become excruciating by bedtime and most of his scheduled medications were drooled out onto his t-shirt, breaking my shattered heart into even smaller bits. Once he laid his handsome head down for the night, I stayed awhile to make sure his breathing was not impaired. He gurgled, grimaced, and coughed a phlegmy cough before eventually drifting off to sleep. I slipped out for a restless night of my own.

I was up before the sun and went right to Billy's room only to find him stumbling around alone in the shadows of dawn with a mouth full of yogurt, oozing with crushed meds, drooling down his chin. He had no eyeglasses to assist him. Where were the caregivers? An electronic mat was promised to set off an alarm when his feet touched the floor, but no one came. The halls were empty and silent. What if I had heeded their suggestion to visit my children in a distant state now that our *new family* had promised to compassionately lighten my burden? The what-ifs flooded my mind—choking, falling, aspiration. Where were all of their promises? Where were the caregivers that Saturday morning?

I cleaned up the love of my life, helped him rinse his mouth, cleaned his stained bottom and his glasses, and dressed him for the day. He relaxed against me and cooperated through obvious discomfort. I left him resting and went to see what should be done about the meds that had been drooled out rather than taken in. I wanted to be sure the new medication had not been mixed into the orange goo dribbling down his chin, but was informed that due to an unfortunate computer glitch, it had been. My anger burned. The what-ifs came back stronger and trust would never be redeemed. It had not even been one month since I locked Billy behind those unsafe walls. They had failed, and failed miserably. They were as dangerous as Billy's monster, but there was nowhere for us to run.

I returned to find him lethargic, twisted with pain, and drooling out any fluid I offered. I slipped on his jacket, wriggled his feet into his tennis shoes and guided him into the car, right past the front desk of our *new family* where no offer of assistance was uttered.

It was the first time Billy had been on the outside in weeks and was too ill to notice. The urgent care office was only a few blocks away and our wait was short to see the doctor on call. A quick assessment and a swab of Billy's mouth revealed a fungal infection that required yet another medication to be crushed into his yogurt. Could it have been a coincidence that this happened after giving him several doses of the new drug? Could his discomfort have been the cause of the monster's raging temper? Why was *I* asking these questions? Why weren't *they*? Why weren't they showing up in his room when his electronic matt was plugged in? I asked them to test it when we returned.

"Oh my goodness, it isn't working," was their surprised response.

How many days had gone by? How many more would have gone by with my Billy fumbling around for the bathroom, or his glasses, or the door if I had not been there? How could I go home and leave him in the hands of under-staffed, non-observant employees? He was the father of my children, and the man who had provided for me for nearly twenty-nine years. I had promised to protect him, and he deserved so much more. Guilt would surely devour me.

The weekend seemed to never end as I sat watching his labored breathing and painful swallowing, waiting for the new anti-fungal medicine to work its magic, and all the while considering a visit to the emergency room. Sunday afternoon had shown some improvement in his ability to swallow. But as evening slipped in, a trip to the restroom where Billy urinated a bowl full of scarlet pee raised my concerns to an even higher level.

He finally slept that night and I was grateful to see Monday morning. I called Billy's primary physician. Dr. T. always told me the hard truth with gentleness and I trusted him. So I was on guard all that day and night when he suggested a trip to the emergency room should Billy deliver more scarlet pee. But by Tuesday morning Billy had not peed at all for far too long, and his sore throat was growing worse again. I slipped on Billy's jacket and shoes, and once again led him past the front desk, through the glass doors and out to the car without a single offer of assistance. I coaxed him through the emergency department doors where we would spend hours waiting for blood-work and x-ray results. The diagnosis included a peritonsillar abscess, dehydration, and low potassium levels due to diarrhea caused by a flare-up of his pesky colitis, brought on by the anti-fungal medication prescribed after our visit to urgent care over the weekend. Could it get much worse? Yes, yes it could.

The pharmacy affiliated with Billy's new home was sent the prescription for antibiotics intended to relieve Billy's discomfort from the serious and extremely painful abscess on his tonsil, but unfortunately they had run out and he would not get his first dose until the following afternoon. Could it get more unbelievable? Of course it could. It had become a sad cartoon and my Billy was paying the price.

By then illness had given the monster unlimited access to Billy's remaining bits, and it began to nibble at his desire to thrive. He ate far less and drank little. The caregivers and I offered, but he mostly refused. We tricked him with finger foods, slipping them between his fingers as he paced, and it worked some of the time, but not often enough. He was fading, weak, his head always drooping, and mostly hurting and afraid. I wrapped his neck in heat throughout the day and massaged the stiffness of his muscles, yet he was still able to lift his head for only moments at a time. Memories of beach walks and gathering sticks flooded my mind. It hadn't been so long ago that he held the elbow of his daughter on her wedding day, battled the waves of a Hawaiian bay, or climbed into the boat for an afternoon of crabbing with Captain George. Anger stood me up tall and I pushed hard against the monster and held on tight to my Billy. I brought his face to mine and repeated again, "I will love you forever, Billy. Remember." He returned a feeble, "I remember."

Thursday morning glimmered with a bit of hope. With antibiotics finally flowing through his veins, Billy began to feel better. He was alert and willing to meet with his psychiatric doctor to discuss his medication regimen. The spring sunshine warmed his face through the car window as we drove slowly through the city, and he relaxed. I reached over and lifted his drooping head so he could enjoy the beauty of the morning. Why couldn't he hold his head up? I asked every doctor we had seen, but it was just another mystery answered with nothing more than a shrug of the shoulders.

We left the psychiatrist's office with a new air of hope. That Nurse had gone with us to explain Billy's aggressive outbursts, and a newly prescribed anti-depressant would solely replace the anti-psychotic and the frightening mood stabilizer that had been added most recently. I was hopeful and tempted his appetite with a cheeseburger before we returned to the monster's cage. He nibbled, weakly, his head hanging low. His eyes met mine after a few small bites and he shook his head. He couldn't finish. I was just happy he tried. We went back and he rested. The hopeful morning quickly faded into a hopeless evening. Billy was again in much pain, holding his back now and unable to pee at all. Kidney stones? Urinary tract infection? We were weary.

The monster joined Billy and me that night and pushed and pulled us through the lobby while our *new family* watched us struggle once again past the front desk, through the glass doors, and out into the dark night on our way to the emergency room, alone with the monster. He continued to push Billy and me around the waiting room. He threatened the nurses, causing the security guard to be on high alert, and it seemed to take forever for the doctor to approve a *calm-him-down-now* pill. Many more hours, hard fought battles, and a painful catheter procedure later, we found ourselves back in the monster's cage with a diagnosis of further dehydration, low potassium due to unrelenting diarrhea, and possible kidney stones. A follow-up with Dr. T was advised.

The following week was riddled with difficult appointments. The monster was uncooperative and paced angrily around examination rooms. Bites of yogurt now overflowed with crushed medication which included an even higher dose of potassium, and Billy's colitis raged. Angry outbursts during clean-ups were frequent and throughout the nighttime hours, he was left unclean most often.

A scheduled visit to the same neurologist's office that had given our monster his name was also difficult, and the new nurse practitioner was astounded at his rapid decline over the past months. He suggested that I join a support group and searched a board covered with notes held up by push-pins for any helpful information, but came up empty. He suggested I search on my own. I wouldn't. I hadn't the time. I did find it odd, though, that a neurologist's office could offer no assistance to the caregiver of the mentally impaired. Awareness slapped me hard on the other cheek.

The latest symptom of urinary retention led us to the office of a compassionate and patient urologist. He was empathetic toward my helplessness and confusion. We discussed, Billy paced. We waited for urine sample and ultrasound results. Billy messed his pants while we waited, and calmly allowed me to clean him. The monster always stepped aside and allowed me to clean my Billy, but battled back when the caregivers came near. Urine results led to another medication. His forced yogurt bites must have tasted terrible.

A bit of light peered through the darkness and glimmered for nearly two weeks. Billy's throat seemed to be healing and he held his head up some. But he would not eat, and he drank so little. The colitis continued to rage and the monster continued to frighten the caregivers during clean-ups. The darkness once again shut out the tiny bit of light when a morning caregiver revealed deep ulcers on Billy's inner thighs, caused by a soiled brief rubbing between his thighs while he had paced throughout the night. That Nurse was summoned. I cleaned him again, put on a fresh brief, and she brought in medicated cream. He grimaced in pain while I did my best to gently slather the freshly cleansed wounds. How did they appear so quickly? Guilt had been woven into my fibers.

I stayed with Billy all day and into the late hours of the evening. I draped a warmed rice bag around his neck while we paced the boring halls. I slipped a plastic water bottle into his fist and guided it to his lips often. We tricked him with pudding and cookies stuffed with his meds; and I showered, shaved, and readied him for bed. His wounds were painful but he let me medicate them. The monster was quiet but not yet sleepy, and with a promise from his caregiver to show him to his bed soon, I left him. I should not have.

I opened the door to the early morning light in Billy's room to find it empty. The bed was still made and everything exactly the way I had left it the night before. I went in search of Billy, and found him drooped in a chair, asleep in the sitting room. The night shift reported that he had spent the wee hours wandering, stopping only for momentary naps on random furniture throughout the unit. The monster had refused their promised attempts at tucking him into bed. But the bed was unrumpled and just as I had left it. More lies? Had they simply dodged the monster all night, leaving my Billy to battle on his own?

I woke him, showered and shaved him, replaced his soiled brief and medicated his wounds. The monster once again quietly stepped aside. The antibiotics had wreaked havoc with his colitis and he had messed his pants several times throughout the day. When was the last dose of antibiotics given? *Had* the last dose been given? How many doses were left before we could calm the colitis? I had asked several times and received no reply. I asked again. The med-tech would check, but never returned. I stayed with Billy the entire day, hoping he would sip water or nibble at a meal. He would do little of either. He was tired. Afternoon slipped into evening as I paced the day away on his elbow. I readied him for bed, brushed his teeth, cleaned his glasses, and medicated his wounds. I looked into his eyes and said again "I will love you forever, Billy. Remember." He did not respond. I prayed that my voice had penetrated the monster's growl and reached my Billy's spirit.

I stayed until the dishes were done, the floors were mopped and the caregivers had reappeared from the laundry room and resident rooms. It was well into the evening when I left Billy wandering the dizzying perimeter of his cage with another promise from his caregiver to tuck him into bed. Surely he would sleep all night. We were both battle weary.

All those I trusted on the outside feared it would be too dangerous to free Billy and fight the monster on my own. Even Dr. T. advised against my threats of escape. The only thing left for me to do was stay with my Billy all day *and* all night. That was my new strategy, before all hell broke loose. And I will forever regret leaving him that final night within the frailty of another promise.

CHAPTER **29**

ALL HELL BROKE LOOSE

HEARTBREAK AND I were snuggled up together under a blanket when That Nurse broke the silence once again, and her frantic tone filled me with panic too. Billy's monster had injured an elderly resident and chaos had shaken the memory care unit. I stepped into the chaos to find Billy pacing wildly in his room. He had messed his pants yet again and was fighting back against the caregivers. My stern command shocked him into stillness. I cleaned him, medicated his wounds and changed his soiled clothes. He was ill, and growing more so.

Explanations void of confirmed fact bounced around the unit. Billy had tried to push through the doorway of the elderly lady's room, injuring her hand, and she had been *escorted* to the emergency room. The monster had been too strong, and help had arrived on the scene too late. Were the halls void of guards at the battle's onset? Where was the caregiver that had promised to tuck Billy into bed that night? Had Billy roamed alone with his monster in a desperate search for the safety of his own room? To Billy all of the doors would look alike.

"How will Billy know which room belonged to him?" Jamie and I had asked Mr. Marketing Director that fateful day barely a month ago.

His confident response was that several caregivers would be *ever-present* and would *frequently* guide him to the safety of his own room. Where were they that night? Perhaps they were folding towels. I should have stayed.

That Nurse had rallied an ally onto the chaotic scene, a large nurse. A hero had been called to command the monster, and the hero's condemning tone set me on edge. The other residents were not safe while the monster roamed free, and Billy's removal would be immediate. Billy was powerless over his monster, and emergency room visits, illness, and medication had left him bound behind the monster's outbursts. He was not well, and I chose the emergency room option over the hero's ridiculous suggestion to have the monster monitored within the confines of a behavioral health facility. Exasperation and I slipped on Billy's jacket and shoes and led him once again through the darkness, *alone*, with no final offer of assistance. Where was *my* hero?

We paced with the monster huffing and puffing throughout the waiting room for what seemed an eternity. The elderly lady emerged from behind secured doors, her hand wrapped in a bandage and her frail arm tucked into the safety of a sling. That Nurse appeared at her side, displaying concern for the elderly lady, but her cloak of compassion was transparent and true motives of self-preservation smoldered beneath it. That Nurse had not shown Billy compassion, and she did not acknowledge us. She could not see past his monster. She may have been warmed by the gentleness of my Billy's spirit had she tried.

Thursday, April the twenty-third, was nearing its end; and I watched as Billy finally slept between the cold metal rails of his new bed, draped in a blanket fresh from the warmer and delivered by a *real* nurse wearing a uniform of *true* compassion.

The *calm-him-down-now* medications had done their job. The nurse had done her job. We were left to wait. Hours had passed when a young doctor finally knocked and pushed through the door. He began a familiar line of questioning directed toward Billy when he began to stir between the rails. Had he not read the chart? *Was* there a chart? I once again stepped in to explain Billy's inability to respond and filled the clueless physician in on the events of the evening. More blood was extracted and equipment attached in hopes of also extracting a urine sample. Just as quickly as he had appeared, the doctor disappeared into the bright lights and bustle of the emergency room, leaving us in shadow again when he pulled the door mostly shut behind him. More waiting. Billy's monster had left him exhausted, and once again he slept. I pulled two stiff plastic chairs together and curled up beneath Billy's flannel shirt. A beam of light peered through the partially open door, and now and then I would catch a glimpse of blue as a nurse scurried past. The room was cold, the chairs were hard, and Billy stirred often.

The black hands of the large white clock that had been tick-tocking throughout the night and into the early morning read five o'clock when another doctor finally burst through the door and jumped right into apologies for our wait and explanations of test results. She sat down on her haunches, looked me directly in the eyes, and melded fact and compassion into her prediction of the monster's consumption of my Billy. It would grow stronger, meaner, and would never be mastered. I needed to prepare for the final battle. She admitted my Billy into the hospital and prescribed a regimen of drugs intended to calm the colitis and allow his body to heal. Until then, a room on the fifth floor would be a temporary cage and new guards would be assigned to his monster.

The new guards would never leave Billy's side. He was now a danger to himself and others. A safety belt was buckled around his waist, tethering him to his newly assigned twenty-four-hour guard. The new guard was patient and paced the shiny, tiled corridor of the fifth floor with Billy and his monster for hours at a time. All of the new guards were fearless and restraining the monster became their top priority. Antipsychotics quickly replaced the recently prescribed antidepressant, and Billy's psychiatrist was immediately replaced with the psychiatrist on staff with the hospital. Relief rode in alongside the strength and kindness of our new army, and made releasing the reins of caregiver and accepting the powerless position of mere visitor, slightly tolerable.

Billy's body responded quickly to the new regimen of medications and without the need for constant battles over clean-ups, the wounds on his inner thighs slowly began to heal. His wrinkled blue hospital gown was often twisted beneath the safety belt fastened around his middle, and in slippered feet he continued to shuffle the corridor's perimeter, at the elbow of a sturdy guard.

The antipsychotics had reduced the monster's temper to a few snorts and growls throughout the weekend, and although Billy was rumpled, scruffy, and tired, he perked up a bit when I entered his room. My heart melted when one gentle guard believed I was able to calm Billy more than the medications, and for me he would nibble a bit at lunch or dinner. Was he still peering out from behind the tangles? Did he know my face? Or *sense* the tugging of our spirits? His body was betraying him far faster than his mind now. Guilt and bewilderment were my undergarments.

By Sunday evening Billy's monster still had not raged, and I left him in the sturdy hands of our new army with a renewed hope for a full night of rest.

CHAPTER 30

A CAGE WITHIN A CAGE

MONDAY MORNING'S SORROW fell like a hammer on Sunday evening's hope. A battle had raged while I slept. The new army did not require my assistance and reinforcements had been summoned. Haldol had been poured into my Billy's veins, and a proper bathroom clean-up completed against his will. He hunched, weary and pale in the dim light of morning, shaky and bedraggled at the bed's rail when I pushed past the heavy door and into the cramped confines of his room. A guard sat silent in a chair and breakfast sat untouched and cold on an uninviting tray. I slipped my arms under his and whispered, "I will love you forever, Billy. Remember." His arms dangled at his side and his chin fell heavy into my shoulder. He was so very battle weary.

I was grateful for my full night of oblivion. It had left me armed and ready to stand strong through new battles waiting at the far end of that long, shiny corridor. A new cage had been prepared for the monster, a cage within a cage, with no route for escape. There would be a frequent changing of the guards, sitting watch behind a long counter, trained to monitor and manage the monster's unwieldly behavior. But in the new cage, Billy slept. Twenty-four hours passed, and still he slept. I sat next to him for bits of time, but he only stirred. Forty-eight hours had gone by before we finally guided him up and onto wobbly legs. He was weak and the new guards walked with him. We tempted him with morsels of meals, and refusals finally led to acceptance of only ice cream and apple juice. I rarely left my Billy and the guards were kind. We paced away the days and late into the evenings, back and forth past the counter of guards, forced to turn at the blockade of locked double doors securing each end of the much shorter, shiny corridor.

Unsavory reactions to the difficulties of life had temporarily landed a circus of unstable roommates into the same cage with Billy and his monster, and they came and went while Billy's body healed. A variety of rounding doctors teamed up to adjust doses of several antipsychotic medications, hoping to temper the monster's unpredictable temper. We paced while acute illness waned. Haldol remained the guards' weapon against the monster's threats and Billy's strength waned too. Forced inward by medication, the monster began to wage war on battlefields we could no longer see. Billy's dull blue eyes were vacant and his body had begun a slow and painful betrayal. He hunched and twitched, pacing at my elbow beneath the heavy weight of fear. I held him long before we turned at each end of the shiny corridor, and he rested against my embrace.

"I will love you forever, Billy. Remember," became my mantra. We cried; the guards watched.

The will to fight back also waned, and the guards allowed me to shower and shave my sweetheart again. Each night I soothed the tremors deep in his muscles and coaxed his contracted legs down onto the mattress beneath several warmed blankets. I fed him ice cream from a plastic spoon and he smiled sometimes. I waited for him to sleep before slipping out each night, and returned each morning prepared for battle.

With the battle of acute illness behind us, the battle for a permanent and safe cage for the monster was underway. Our *family* at the memory care unit was eager to disown us and willingly released us from the clutches of their incompetency, but my Billy would never again be free. Awareness was about to give me a painful black eye.

The business end had little compassion for the human end and Billy's discharge from the hospital was looming. He needed a new home, but fear of the monster brought rejection. Not enough time had passed since the last battle, and more time was needed to prove that the monster had turned its fury to Billy's interior.

Awareness had clenched its fist, ready to strike, when Dr. Psychologist strolled in wearing a sport coat reeking of arrogance. He had been tasked with the nasty business of delivering a remedy to our conundrum. The remedy Dr. Psychologist pulled from his collection of worthless remedies? Admittance to the state mental hospital for the remainder of Billy's life. Awareness let me have it, a painful right jab, leaving behind a black eye that would never fully heal.

"But Billy's mind cannot be *counseled*, it is dissolving, bit by bit, with each passing moment," was my exasperated response.

My rambling fell upon deaf ears. Dr. Psychologist was steadfast in his remedy and attempted to calm my fears with a vague description of the Alzheimer's unit located within a secure wing of the state hospital. His daft remedy left *him* appearing as impaired as those he treated, and far meaner than Billy's monster. He became an instant adversary in my war, a traitor and a spy.

I recruited Jamie, Levi, and Autumn in my search. Our community and our state had abandoned us, and Dr. Psychologist had tried to cover their shortcomings. They could not offer a safe haven for my Billy while the monster stormed the tangled, war-torn fields of his mind, in preparation for its final victory. Perhaps there were faraway places with braver soldiers, and for days we frantically searched while Billy grew weaker. I stumbled through a cloud of panic, my black eye swelling more with each rejection. I began to pray for the war's end.

The rapid and steady betrayal of Billy's physical body confounded me, and I jumped back into the tunnel of independent research. Tremors, contractions, and twitches seemed odd symptoms of Alzheimer's and left me desperately searching for answers that might explain Billy's most recent agony. A similar story finally caught my attention, the painful symptoms and rapid progression nearly identical to my Billy's. I printed off the lengthy, detailed story and submitted it to the guards.

I recognized the tall, soft-spoken doctor who returned with the story in hand just a few days later. He had read it, *at home*, and would recommend a new evaluation of Billy by the hospital's neurologist. A spark of compassion kindled a new flame of hope, unsure of what I was hoping for.

A quick assessment of Billy's tremors, twitches, and painful contractions, along with his dull and unresponsive gaze, made the neurologist's diagnosis of Multiple System Atrophy instantly apparent to his trained eye. Billy's monster was possibly far more complex than we had known, and had discreetly ravaged far more than his beautiful mind since that cold day in January three years ago. While I had been searching for Billy amongst a diversion of twisted tangles, the monster had been pausing the music of his heart, tugging at his muscles, blurring his vision, and roaring him into silence. Billy had been left with little will or strength. The war was very near its end and a safe haven had, *so far,* eluded us.

CHAPTER 31

SURRENDER

THE SOFT-SPOKEN DOCTOR gently offered an alternative to Dr. Psychologist's ridiculous remedy.

"Hospice," he whispered, "Comfort care. They will help Billy rest...and sleep."

Sleep. They would help him sleep. No further hope for moments of clarity. It was time to surrender. For my Billy. He was thin and frail, and a safe haven would finally welcome him. Just a few more days of quiet battle would ensure his release.

Levi's final year of medical school had come to a close and *my* hero soon rode in to lift the fatigue of battle. He brought laughter, took the elbow of his father while we strolled the shiny corridor, and helped me navigate the steady flow of medical jargon. Judi and Tammy brought more laughter and strolled with Billy too. He smiled and strolled, took bits of ice cream and napped. Those were our final days in the cage.

Monday, the eighteenth of May, brought the official day of surrender. Sunshine lit up the morning and Billy's face when we wheeled him out the front doors of the hospital and into the freshness of spring. He knew the freshness and his eyes smiled. The monster had bound his body and his mind, but his spirit tasted freedom.

The safe haven waited. A large, open room, hosting another bed with metal rails in the center. A sofa and a recliner for waiting, sat beneath windows that sucked in sunshine and camouflaged the darkness of war. A door opened to a sunlit patio where more waiting furniture sat hauntingly empty, and a sea of thick green grass bumped up to spring blossoms, adding color to Billy's new haven. He stood hunched and silent at Levi's side, peering at the outside world through the glass in the door.

It had been weeks since the sunshine warmed him and he drank in the scent of the earth. Levi and I led him through the sea of green in a fresh hospital gown and slippers, and I watched fear fall away from his face. He relaxed against the strength of his son's grip. He was safe. He felt it.

Many were preparing to miss him and popped in and out of the quiet room. Billy's Aunt Mary sat in quiet comfort often. Judi and Tammy held his hand a final time, and Levi slept on the waiting sofa every night, easing Billy's confusion when he stirred in the shadows. The gentle angels of hospice floated in and out with magical potions that quieted the remaining rumbles of the monster and calmed his body's steady betrayal. Levi and I waited, in the waiting furniture. Billy slept often, and then more often.

Saturday morning had left me on my own again. Levi's graduation ceremony from medical school was to be held at nine o'clock in the morning on the twenty-seventh day of May, and it called him away. He would not see his father again and he shared his parting prayer with me. In the silent shadows on the waiting sofa he had prayed that his father's spirit would be set free in time to join him as he walked before his peers to receive his diploma. I prayed The Taker would answer his prayer.

Billy stirred less, and then much less. And that Saturday morning just hours after Levi had gone, a final stirring pulled him deep into the in-between. No more walks, no more ice-cream, only sleep. Withering sleep. The magic potions had washed away the agony, the monster had claimed the spoils of war, and The Taker had sent Azrael. The spirit world beckoned my Billy, and for days he faded further into the in-between.

I was on my own for just one day. Autumn floated in and her steady spirit steadied me. She is the peace of Sunday, and she arrived on Sunday. My guardian had replaced my hero and her reserve of strength would gently carry me over the threshold of war. We pulled the waiting furniture up close to Billy and waited through each night. We held his hands, I on one side, she on the other. We kissed his cheeks. We waited in the waiting furniture on the sunny patio each afternoon. He slept. We wept. And waited.

Tuesday evening slowly faded into the still dark hours of Wednesday, the twenty-seventh day of May. The hands of the clock that had been tick-tock-ing throughout the night and into the early hours of morning read five o'clock when Billy's baby girl reached across his motionless chest to squeeze my hand.

"It's time, Mama," she whispered. "It's been more than a minute."

The orchestra had set down their instruments, silencing the symphony one final time. I had closed my eyes and missed the final rise and fall of my Billy's chest. Autumn had not, and she alone holds the memory of her daddy's final breath in the stillness of a dark spring morning in May.

At The Taker's command, Azrael led my Billy out of the in-between and beyond the veil. He was finally free. Free to be with Levi on his graduation day only hours later.

CHAPTER **32**

FOR BILLY

IT RAINED. HEAVEN and my heart shed tears for days. May slipped into June and preparations to celebrate your short life began. June the twenty-first, Father's Day, the only day Levi's unforgiving schedule would allow, was reserved for a final party in your honor. You loved parties, Billy, and we would party for you. With you. One more time.

A wall of windows facing the western sky overlooked the mighty Missouri River and lit up the large banquet room. Long tables dressed in crisp white linen held steaming silver pots filled with savory pork sitting next to mountains of dinner rolls and giant bowls of potato salad. Colorful trays of fruit shimmered next to bottles of red wine, and trays of brightly colored cupcakes adorned with plastic fish sat waiting at the end. Double doors led to an outdoor deck that sat high above a pond leading up to acres of rolling green glistening with the freshness of spring, and oversized coolers stuffed with ice and beer waited along the deck's perimeter.

Memories were set to music, and rows of stark white chairs began to fill with those lucky enough to have shared a snapshot of time with you. Words meant for comfort poured over our loved ones, and pierced my selfish heart. You are in a better place, young and free. I should find comfort in that. Perhaps in time, I will.

Tears were dried and paper plates overflowing with colorful buffet were devoured in the warm sunshine. Your life's celebration flowed with beer and laughter and your name could be heard bouncing amongst those already missing your gentle uniqueness. Family was gathered, a group here, a group there, and photos were taken. Levi and Autumn were uncomfortable in their mortal skins, and struggled to meld celebration with sorrow. The three of us were gathered. We stood tall and proud, dressed all in black, smiling through tears beneath the brilliant blue of a Montana sky in June.

I will love you forever, Billy. Remember.

www.ingramcontent.com/pod-product-compliance
Lightning Source LLC
Chambersburg PA
CBHW020517100426
42813CB00030B/3278/J